BACK TO
Active

HOW TREATING HEARING LOSS & TINNITUS
can change your **life**, maintain your **independence**,
and may reduce your risk of **dementia**

Dr. Al Turri, AuD
Dr. Keith N. Darrow, PhD

Back to Active: How Treating Hearing Loss & Tinnitus Can Change Your Life, Maintain Your Independence, and May Reduce Your Risk of Dementia — by Dr. Al Turri, AuD, and Dr. Keith N. Darrow, PhD

Project Director: Jared M. Brader, MBA
Editor: Kelly Martin
Graphics: Steve Ruesch
Interior Design: Five J's Design, FiveJsDesign.com

First Printing: September 2017
Second Printing: August 2018
Third Printing: December 2019

ISBN: 978-1-70563-660-2

Thanks & Acknowledgments

Christiane C. Turri, my wife, best friend and incredible mother of our three daughters. Without you there is no me, thank you for being my example daily on how to live for something bigger than myself. Your faith and desire to walk in the light daily has inspired me more than you will ever know. Eu te amo Christiane!

A special thanks to my parents, **Al and Mary Lou**. Dad worked two jobs for most of my childhood and his example instilled in me his fierce work ethic and the mind set that work is over when the job is done right. Mom always made due with what she had and made everything she had seem like more than what she needed. I thank my mom for my never ending optimism and belief that I have everything I need to be successful.

Michelle Menendez, Au.D., my clinical fellow supervisor at Baypines VA taught me that you're never wrong doing right by the patient, regardless of what policy you navigate around or what it costs in resources and time.

The Villages Health System for allowing me to create the most incredible practice setting for an audiologist: Primary care physicians and audiologists working shoulder-to-shoulder with amazing resources and a shared goal of taking care of the whole patient.

Keith Darrow, Ph.D., thank you for allowing me to collaborate with you and to join your crusade of striving for excellence in audiology.

Nora Stewart, M.S., thank you for helping me find my why again! Thank you for Entheos Audiology Cooperative, Hearing the Call and hearing smiles.

Table of Contents

BACK TO
Active

Preface

Today, approximately 48 million people in the United States are suffering from hearing loss. Yet, nearly 40 million of them go without treatment. Hence, the reason I wrote this book.

- *Do you want to remain independent and live an active life as you age?*

- *Did you know that hearing problems, even at the mildest stage, can lead to social isolation and increase the risk of dementia?*

- *Do you or a loved one have impaired hearing?*

I'm Dr. Keith N. Darrow, Ph.D. CCC-A, a trained Neuroscientist and practicing Clinical Audiologist. If you or a loved one has answered yes to any of the above questions, I encourage you to read this book and learn how you can live a better, more active, more engaged, and healthier life as you age. For over twenty years, I have been helping my patients, and their loved ones, break free of their hearing loss and live an active, engaged life—free of the worry, stress, and medical consequences of untreated hearing loss.

Hearing is what connects us to others. Hearing is a requirement for every personal and professional relationship we have; it is the building block of communication.

Hearing is also one of the major senses; in fact, I believe it is the single most important sense we have. While hearing certainly plays a major role in our fight or flight, prey vs. predator, and history as human beings, hearing today has the important role of keeping us communicating and connected with the world around us—at home, at work, and in our community. To further support my claim that hearing is the single most important sense we have, I offer the fact that the organ of hearing, the cochlea (AKA the inner ear), is embedded deep in the hardest bone in the entire human body, the petrous portion of the temporal bone (i.e. petrous means "stone/rock")—thus providing our organ of hearing significant protection.

I have put together this book to help you understand the dire consequences of untreated hearing loss and to introduce you to how today's medical options for treating hearing loss can not only help improve hearing, but also improve cognitive function, decrease your risk of developing dementia, depression, and falling, while also increasing your physical activity, and helping you live a happier and healthier lifestyle as you actively age.

Hearing loss has been listed by the Department of Health and Human Services as the third most common chronic health condition affecting seniors. *Third!* Hearing loss is estimated to affect nearly 50% of adults between the age of sixty to seventy years young, nearly 2/3 of adults between seventy to eighty years young, and the numbers only go up from there! As we live longer and science continues to increase life expectancy, we need to be best prepared to deal with this debilitating disorder and understand how it can impact our lives.

My journey up to this point has been filled with over twenty years of experience—from student to clinician to scientist to college professor and back to clinician and patient advocate. I was lucky to discover what I love to do in life, and as a result I have the good fortune to work with patients and their families every day as they embark on the journey of improved hearing and clarity.

While my elementary and high school performance wasn't much to speak of (in fact, I was dismissed from high school twice—but that is a story for a different day!), once I found my path of helping people understand and improve the process of communication in their daily lives, it all became incredibly easy for me.

In fact, I was on the Dean's List nearly every semester in college, graduated in the top 5% of my Clinical Audiology Program in New York City, and went on to be the only practicing audiologist to complete a Doctoral Degree in the Neuroscience track at M.I.T. and Harvard Medical School.

As a trained Neuroscientist, expert in Speech and Hearing Bioscience and Technology, and a practicing clinical audiologist, I have a unique perspective on how the brain works and how hearing relates to overall health, well-being, and cognitive function. I also understand how treating hearing loss *early* (even before it becomes a problem that you and everybody around you can notice) significantly impacts your overall health and cognitive function and how it may significantly reduce your risk of developing dementia.

I believe that I am blessed to have the capability of transforming lives and families every single day. Treating hearing loss is not magic—it is the perfect mix of science and experience, which allows myself and my team to use advances in medical treatment of hearing loss, NeuroTechnology™, to stimulate the brain, improve cognitive function and mental health, and help adults remain independent. And the best part—it is simple for patients to manage and it's affordable!

"I treat every patient like family and if I wouldn't do it for my mom or dad then I don't do it for a patient. Hearing, like life itself, is a precious gift. It deserves special care."

Dr. Al Turri, Au.D., is the Director of Audiology for The Villages Health, where he leads a team of six audiologists dedicated to serving America's Healthiest Hometown® through the comprehensive education, diagnosis and treatment of hearing loss. Dr. Turri joined The Villages Health in 2011 to establish the Audiology department, bringing with him deep experience in patient care, hearing aid technology and operational management.

Dr. Turri began his career in the medical field in 1997 after selling a wholesale/retail flower business. While pursuing a master's degree in speech-language pathology, he was required to shadow audiologists in a clinical setting. Upon experiencing a patient's response to a proper hearing aid fitting, he changed his course of study to audiology and never looked back.

Dr. Turri earned a master's degree in Audiology from the University of South Florida in 2001 and a doctoral degree from the Pennsylvania College of Optometry School of Audiology in 2006. He was selected for a coveted clinical fellowship at Bay Pines VA Healthcare Systems, where he completed his internship/residency fitting hearing aids and providing aural rehabilitation.

Following his clinical fellowship, Dr. Turri worked in a variety of audiology settings in several states, including medical clinics, hearing aid manufacturing and operations management. He returned to Florida in 2007 and opened an audiology practice inside of a primary care physician office, launching his entrepreneurial venture of what was to become Harmony Hearing Centers of America. Dr. Turri grew Harmony into nine locations throughout Central Florida, delivering close to

2,000 hearing aids per year. Eager to shift his focus back to patient care, he sold the business in 2015 and joined The Villages Health full-time.

In addition to working side-by-side with primary care physicians to serve patients at The Villages Health, Dr. Turri dedicates his time and passion to Hearing the Call, a nonprofit organization supported by Entheos Audiology Cooperative that provides aid to people without access to audiology care throughout the world. Following a humanitarian trip to South Africa, he established a local give-back program, supported by The Villages Health and Hearing the Call, to help Central Florida residents in need to gain access to hearing healthcare.

Dr. Turri is a Fellow of the Academy of Doctors of Audiology and the Florida Academy of Audiology. He is ABA Board Certified in Audiology and is a Certified Dementia Risk Educator for the American Brain Council. Dr. Turri and his wife, Christiane, have three daughters.

Education

2006 Doctor of Audiology
Pennsylvania College of Optometry School of Audiology
2001 Master of Science, Audiology
University of South Florida, Tampa
1992 Bachelor of Science, Social Sciences
University of South Florida, Tampa

Professional Affiliations and Certifications

- Academy of Doctors of Audiology | *Fellow*
- Florida Academy of Audiology | *Fellow*
- ABA Board Certification | *Audiology*
- American Brain Council | *Certified Dementia Risk Educator*
- State of Florida Licensed Audiologist AY-1186

Dr. Keith N. Darrow, PhD, is an expert in Speech and Hearing Bioscience and Technology with a doctoral degree from the joint Massachusetts Institute of Technology (M.I.T) and Harvard Medical School program. He is a former Clinical Professor at Northeastern University (Boston, MA) and is currently a tenured professor at Worcester State University.

Dr. Darrow's clinical experience is vast and includes a clinical fellowship at the Department of Otolaryngology at Brigham and Women's Hospital (Boston, MA) and a trainingship at the Audiology Department in the East Orange (NJ) Veterans Association Hospital. He is the owner of the Hearing and Balance Centers of New England and founder of the Healthy Hearing Foundation of New England, as well as a board member of the Sound of Life Foundation (both non-profit organizations dedicated to providing education and hearing health care for those in need). He was recently named the Director of Audiology Research at Intermountain Audiology and has chosen to lead the Excellence In Audiology movement across the country.

Dr. Darrow is a nationally recognized speaker, trainer, and researcher and has been conducting research at the Massachusetts Eye and Ear Infirmary for over fifteen years. His publications and research have been cited over 550 times. On a personal note, Dr. Darrow and his wife Laura have three children (Ella, Mae and Charlie) who love to ski and travel to National Parks together. He also serves on the board of directors for the Worcester County Reserve Deputy Sheriffs Association and provides countless hours of volunteer service in his communities.

Foreword

Hearing Health Care is Total Health Care

While pursuing a master's degree in speech-language pathology, I was required to shadow audiologists in a clinical setting. I will never forget the day I saw a patient respond to a proper hearing aid fitting. It was life-changing—for the patient *and* me.

That day, I changed the course of my study to audiology—and that decision altered the course of my career and my life.

I started what would become Harmony Hearing Centers of America where each year I helped more than 2,000 people receive a proper fitting for hearing aids and instantly improved their quality of life.

Many people ask why I chose to leave a lucrative private practice for a career at The Villages Health. After all, I was fulfilling my true passion in life of helping people improve their hearing health, enhance their lifestyle, and reduce their risk of cognitive decline. I was living the dream—or so I thought.

When I learned about the vision of The Villages Health, I knew I had to be a part of this truly remarkable medical care model where primary care physicians and audiologists work shoulder-to-shoulder to care for the whole patient—not just *hearing* healthcare, but *total* health care.

A New Kind of Health Care Delivery Model

In the Villages®, located in Central Florida, residents live in a unique retirement community, and their health care delivery model is no exception. The Villages Health is specifically designed to fit their active lifestyle. From little to no wait times, to longer appointments with their doctor, everything revolves around the patient's comfort, convenience and care, so they can enjoy this wonderful community and lifestyle for years to come.

In fact, the vision of The Villages Health is to make The Villages and surrounding community America's Healthiest Hometown®. This is accomplished by providing comprehensive health and wellness services and resources that keep people healthy and heal people quickly. For example, doctors at The Villages Health have 50% fewer patients when compared to other physician groups. This allows doctors to spend more time to care for their patients without feeling rushed or running late to the next patient appointment. Likewise, 24/7 urgent care services are provided to patients so they can receive continuity of care from their own provider team at an affordable cost even when they experience a sudden injury or illness. It's incredible!

As a result of their unique model that revolves around the patients' needs, The Villages Health is the number one physician group in North and Central Florida and ranks in the top one percent of the nation's health systems when compared to The Healthcare Effectiveness Data and Information Set (HEDIS), a tool developed by the National Committee for Quality Assurance (NCQA) that's used by more than 90 percent of America's health plans to measure the level of care and service.

The Villages Health is a multi-specialty group. We are comprised of more than 500 employees with over 70 physicians, and 15 different specialties (including audiology). That means when a patient has a major health care concern, their primary care physician can coordinate their care with a specialist like me.

For instance, if one of our primary care physicians' notices that one of their patients is speaking too loudly or having trouble hearing, they don't send them to a hearing aid dispensary down the road. No! Instead, they walk them down the hall to my office so I can effectively evaluate their hearing loss.

Together as a team, we serve more than 52,000 patients in eight locations. It's a dream come true.

The Villages Health has allowed me to build a patient-centered audiology department that provides the highest caliber of licensed audiologists, state-of-the-art diagnostics, and technologically advanced treatment solutions. We are your local source for the comprehensive education, diagnosis, and treatment of hearing loss in The Villages and surrounding community. Plus, I get to do all of this while giving back to the community through Hearing the Call, a nonprofit organization that provides aid to people without access to audiology care, supported by Entheos Audiology Cooperative. This means I help people with a financial need gain access to properly fitted hearing aids.

Now do you understand why I had to be a part of this unique and remarkable health care delivery model?

The Hearing Health Care Approach

Another thing I love about working at The Villages Health is the dedication to health and wellness education. Last year, we offered over 1,500 free educational classes to the community, and we expect to do even more this year.

Many of those classes were about audiology and hearing health. Why? We believe an educated patient ultimately makes better choices, and better choices lead to better outcomes for the patient—you.

Our commitment to education is also why we chose to write this book. We want you to make the best decision for your hearing health.

It can be hard for audiologists like me to get the educational materials to you because we compete with a lot of retail hearing aid stores. These stores take a sales approach, not a health care approach.

The sales approach is what you see most often in the marketplace. Just check the newspaper any Monday and you'll see what I mean. It's hearing aid ad day, and just about every sales tactic you can imagine is represented. This costs a small fortune and contributes significantly to the cost of care for patients.

Many times, these ads promise you a low-cost, high-tech hearing aid. When you respond to the ad, oftentimes the salesperson (not the doctor) whom you wind up in front of is doing his or her best to move the conversation away from the cheap advertised hearing aid to the more expensive one with all the bells and whistles. The problem is that the salesperson doesn't even know if you need that level of technology—or worse, they may not even know how to program those hearing aids so you can achieve your fullest hearing potential.

Another scenario is that you wind up in a hearing aid store that is owned or funded by a hearing aid manufacturer. That means they only sell one brand, and therefore, you will only be fitted with that brand. Unfortunately, not every patient can be fit well with all manufacturers. However, if one manufacturer is the only choice available, then that is the only choice at that location.

In both scenarios, at the end of the experience, you will most likely end up with ITD hearing aids.

Do you have ITD hearing aids or know someone that does? What's an ITD hearing aid, you ask?

An ITD hearing aid is a hearing aid that was purchased, but eventually, they wound up in the drawer. "In The Drawer". ITD.

When this happens, the person with the ITD hearing aids will swear up and down that hearing aids don't work, they cost too much, and they're useless! They could spend the rest of their life thinking there is no help for them when in fact, there *is* help.

When you meet with me and my team, the experience is much different. We take a health care approach because we are health care providers. We are licensed audiologists who are highly trained and motivated to fit you with the hearing aid that is best for your hearing health. We are not salespeople compensated by commission, nor are we committed to any one brand. We are doctors. Your health and wellness are our number one priority. This makes all the difference.

Let me explain more.

Experience the Difference in Hearing Health Care

As you'll read in this book, hearing loss is a progressive, degenerative disorder that not only requires accurate diagnosis, but also ongoing management. It is a serious health concern, and not just anyone is cut out to manage it.

Currently, within the surrounding area of The Villages there are over 40 hearing aid salespeople and nine licensed audiologists. Six of those audiologists work with me at The Villages Health (myself included), two audiologists work for the VA health clinic, and one audiologist works with the local ENT office.

All this to say that if you answer an ad in the paper or stop in a local big box store for a free hearing test, then you are sitting with a hearing aid salesperson, and not a Doctor of Audiology.

Doctors of Audiology have eight years of college education, including four years in a graduate program that includes an intense fourth-year residency.

Individuals selling hearing aids in a retail store typically train on the job, have no graduate training in audiology, and come from a sales background.

I don't know about you, but I would much rather see a doctor, someone with an advanced degree and training, for my medical condition—not a salesperson.

What frequently happens on the retail side is that patients are fit with hearing aids and told to call if they are having any problems. This is less than adequate for the patient to adjust to their new hearing aids.

Instead, patients should be seen weekly early in the process, or at least biweekly, to allow for adaption, tweaking, and assistance with proper use. Once the patient has adapted well to amplification and has demonstrated consistent use, then they should be seen every four to six months for routine maintenance, as well as for programming adjustments based on performance-related outcomes.

The Villages Health Audiology patients have this type of experience—and more.

After being fitted with hearing aids, before you leave the office you will be immediately scheduled for your follow-up appointments.

In addition to the appointments scheduled early in the process, you will also need routine service. That is because your hearing and hearing performance will change over time. By scheduling consistent appointments two to three times per year, we can catch little things before they become big things. This ensures the optimal performance of your technology.

The other issue that arises in a retail model is that the hearing aid specialist is frequently compensated via commission as opposed to a salary. If they don't sell you a hearing aid, then they do not earn any income for the time spent with you. This simply creates a conflict of interest—and that is not in the best interest of the patient.

Every audiologist at The Villages Health gets a paycheck, whether they help you start treatment or not.

Our primary focus is educating you regarding your hearing loss, its implication on your daily life, and the long-term effects on you.

Secondly, and just as important, our function is to assist you with starting treatment and ensuring the best possible outcome for you today and throughout your life. This begins with making sure you understand the significance of your hearing loss and how it impacts your daily life.

Thirdly, the next step is to understand your lifestyle and your individual needs as it relates to your communication needs.

Finally, we select a technology and ensure that you understand that its use is a priority for your total health and well-being.

This hearing health care approach is what you will experience when you meet with an audiologist at The Villages Health.

What to Expect in Your First Appointment?

When you meet with an audiologist with The Villages Health, we will do both a hearing and lifestyle assessment.

You will receive a simple pass/fail hearing screening. If you fail the screening, this could indicate a hearing loss and the next step is to take a comprehensive diagnostic evaluation. This test examines your hearing threshold, your speech discrimination, and your air and bone conduction. These three types of hearing tests allow us to determine whether you have hearing loss, what type of hearing loss you may have and to what degree, and what type of treatment you may need.

We will explain your test results and discuss your treatment options which may include hearing aids. If that is the case, we have a variety of brands that we can work with—and we will find a hearing aid solution that works best for your personal needs so you can improve your hearing and get back to your active lifestyle.

If you are a candidate for hearing aids, you can rest assured that you will receive a risk-free, 30-day trial. This means you can try out your hearings aids to make sure you have the perfect fit *before* committing. During your trial, we will meet often to make necessary adjustments and offer you a 100% money-back guarantee to ensure your complete satisfaction and total hearing health.

After your trial, we will continue to follow up every four months to ensure you experience optimum hearing in all areas of your life. During this time, we will clean your hearing aids, test them to make sure they are working properly, and adjust your programming as needed.

Hearing changes over time, so we will continually assess and adjust your hearing aids. We want you to hear and experience everything at its best, from the TV in your living room and phone calls with grandchildren, to live entertainment or the faint rustling of leaves.

When do you need to see an ENT?

In our classes, we educate patients on anatomy and physiology of the hearing system. We hit home that a large majority of patients in need of hearing health care have what is called "sensorineural" hearing loss, or damage to the inner ear, for which hearing aids are the indicated treatment. Obviously, some cases require surgical intervention. That small percentage of patients are referred to ear, nose, and throat (ENT) physicians for care.

In most cases, patients with hearing loss do *not* require an ENT as part of their care plan, which is another reason we created the hearing health care model of audiology at The Villages Health.

Prior to audiology being onsite in primary care, patients with complaints of hearing loss would have to be referred to an ENT for a consult. After waiting several weeks for an appointment, the ENT upon visual inspection of the ear and learning that the complaint was hearing loss related, would send the patient to their audiologist down the hall.

The patient returns to the ENT post-hearing test only to be informed that they have a hearing loss and need to be rescheduled with audiology to discuss treatment.

This process, in addition to being inefficient, also adds significant cost to the process of delivering hearing health care. Since less than six percent of patients with hearing loss actually have a condition that can be treated by an ENT, the hearing health care model at The Villages Health increases access to care, while simultaneously reducing the cost of overall care.

In The Villages Health model, the patient sees the audiologist first, and if the patient is in that six percent group that requires an ENT, then they are referred accordingly to the appropriate specialist.

Now Let's Get You Back to Active

If hearing loss is holding you back from doing the things you love, spending time with the ones you love, or living the lifestyle you've always dreamed of, then I implore you to schedule an appointment with a licensed audiologist as soon as possible.

If you wait to treat your hearing loss, it can have long-term and potentially devastating effects that reach far beyond lifestyle issues.

A joint study by John Hopkins Medicine and the National Institute on Aging has released powerful data showing untreated hearing loss results in a higher incidence of early-onset dementia. **The #1, single most modifiable factor for reducing the risk of cognitive decline and dementia is the treatment of hearing loss.**

Yes, reducing obesity, diabetes, and/or cardiovascular disease is important. It is also important to increase social activity, enhance your education, and supplement your nutrition. These can all play a part in helping us to reduce the risk of Dementia—and we certainly offer free classes on all of these risk factors as well—but none of these factors, even when combined, are nearly as effective as the treatment of hearing loss.

If you delay treatment, then brain function and cognitive ability can be impaired significantly from auditory deprivation, as well as the cognitive overload caused by reduced hearing.

I promise to educate you on the latest hearing aid technologies (some are nearly invisible), and most importantly, the evidence-based research that will help you make an informed decision about your hearing health. My team and I are dedicated to providing trusted, compassionate care and practical solutions designed to help you achieve hearing clarity, improve brain health and enjoy life to the fullest.

Cheers to your active lifestyle!

Sincerely,

Al Turri, Au.D.

Introduction

The Top 5 Reasons People Avoid Seeing a Hearing Care Specialist

My name is Dr. Keith N. Darrow, and I'm a trained Neuroscientist and Clinical Audiologist! When people hear what I do for a living, they almost automatically...wince! They try not to be too obvious about it. (Hey, I have feelings, too!). It's okay; I'm used to it. The fact is, the less you know about audiology and treating hearing loss, the more reason you have to be afraid of it. Once upon a time, audiology meant one thing: big, heavy, ugly "beige bananas" to be worn on your ear to make sounds louder.

They were hard to put on, hard to make adjustments to, and, frankly, they were pretty terrible at doing anything other than making all sounds louder...this includes speech, background noise, loud ventilation machines, dogs barking, plates clanging, etc.!

For the majority of patients, wearing an old fashioned hearing aid meant avoiding certain social situations, restaurants, family gatherings, playing with grandchildren, etc. Many people still cling to the unfounded notion that all hearing aids are created equal and perform the same way they did back in 1982!

The fact of the matter is that audiology and the clinical science of treating hearing loss is more than just hearing aids. How much more? *Audiology and the medical treatment of hearing loss is devoted to restoring an individual's clarity, restoring personal independence, improving cognitive function and mental health, and addressing the cognitive aspects of hearing loss that can increase the risk of developing dementia.*

Maintaining proper hearing and cognitive health has a significant impact on an individual's life—including all of his or her family, friends, and community members. Properly stimulating cognitive function and maintaining connections from the ear to the brain goes a long way in keeping a patient mentally competent, helping the patient remain autonomous, and helping keep at bay the mind-robbing diseases associated with cognitive decline (i.e. Alzheimer's). Treating hearing loss is a wonderful investment with life-long returns, and yet people still fear walking into a hearing health care provider's office for one simple reason—fear of the unknown!

Hey—it's okay to be worried about the unknown. We all have our reasons for avoiding the doctor. For example, I underwent aggressive management of atypical moles on my body (to avoid potentially pre-cancerous melanoma). I was scared. I avoided starting the treatment for several years. Until I realized that enough is enough…and I had my family bugging me to do something before it was too late. Starting treatment was the right thing to do, and while it was impossible to know the results had I not started treatment…the potential is there for me not having ever had the opportunity to write this book (if you catch my drift!).

For many, visiting a Doctor of Audiology is accompanied by many fears and anxieties. And for each patient, the experience is personal. There are reasons that patients typically wait seven years before being seen by a Doctor of Audiology and beginning treatment of their hearing loss. This list, *Top 5 Reasons People Avoid Seeing a Hearing Care Specialist,* has the most common conversations I have had with patients over the past twenty years about what took them so long to come in to my office.

While you may not place treating potentially pre-cancerous moles and treating hearing loss on the same level of importance, I promise that by the time you are done with this book you will understand why that premise is absolutely wrong and how the consequences of untreated hearing loss can negatively impact every part of your life, even rendering you dependent on others and at a significantly increased risk of developing dementia.

REASON #1 — The Patient Already Knows the Diagnosis Before He or She Ever Steps Foot in the Door.

Individuals with hearing loss have a tendency to wait nearly seven years before raising their hand and admitting they have a problem. Or perhaps it takes a family member nearly seven years to push his or her loved one through our office door! Either way, seven seems to be the "unlucky" number—I say "unlucky" because chances are very high that by the seventh year of experiencing the symptoms of hearing loss, significant damage has been done to the auditory system, which can lower treatment outcomes. I try to explain to all of my patients that hearing loss is a progressive degenerative disorder with neurologic involvement which undoubtedly requires early intervention. In lay terms, that simply means that your hearing will continue to degrade as you age, and the key to maintaining clarity and a higher level of hearing function (i.e. hearing in noisy environments) is to *"catch it early and treat it early."*

I have empathy for the new patient who comes to my office to get his or her first hearing evaluation since grade school because I know, as does the patient, what the results will likely be. It is very brave for a patient to knowingly enter a medical office with the understanding that he or she is likely to receive the diagnosis of progressive degenerative age-related hearing loss. And that this disorder is neither reversible, nor is there a cure. However, there are restorative treatments available that can help the patient stay connected at home, at work, and in the community, and that can help stimulate the brain, improve cognitive function, and even reduce the risk of developing dementia (more on the connections of hearing loss and dementia later in the book!).

REASON #2 — The Patient is Not Sure of His or Her Insurance Coverage for the Procedures and Treatments Involved with Hearing Loss.

Regardless of when you read this book and which administration is running our country, insurance is a complex world to attempt to muddle through, and when it comes to hearing health care coverage, it can be even more murky. BUT…nearly every insurance company I have come across allows for coverage of one hearing evaluation per year by a trained hearing health care specialist (and more testing can be covered if medically necessary, i.e. if the patient notices a significant sudden change in hearing). A hearing evaluation is often considered "preventative" and, in many cases, does not require a referral from your physician.

While it is nearly impossible to speak for every patient and every insurance plan, this is intended to help ease the stress of navigating the process of hearing health care coverage. In fact, I believe any reputable hearing health care practice will have a deep understanding of the insurance regulations in its area and will be able to readily answer any questions you may have about your insurance coverage—or at least be willing to help you find the answer.

In my twenty years of experience in the hearing health care field, I have watched first hand as patient benefits for treatment of hearing loss have evolved—fortunately, in a direction that benefits the patient. Yes, medical treatment of your hearing loss may have an out-of-pocket cost associated with it, but I have seen insurance cover anywhere from 10% to 100% of the costs. And even if you were in the position of having 0% insurance coverage, treating hearing loss can be affordable—and you will learn throughout this book that treating hearing loss is truly priceless and can hardly be assigned a monetary value.

REASON #3 — Patients are Afraid of Being Sold Something.

It's like magic—once you turn the respectful age of sixty, you notice that the content of your mailbox seems to change. Nearly every week, perhaps a few times a week, you are "blessed" (I'm being sarcastic!) to have a full mailbox (both your physical and electronic mailbox) with literature about "essential vitamins for seniors," "how to choose the right assisted living residence," "how to invest your retirement money," "join AARP," and "which digital technology widget is best for your hearing loss." Somewhere along the line, hearing health care started down the dangerous road of becoming a retail transaction. Heck, I've even seen some hearing widgets sold at big-box retailers and chain pharmacies…although I don't know who would ever consider buying medical treatment for a progressive degenerative disorder alongside a giant vat of peanut butter! Like I ask my patients: "*Would you get your colonoscopy performed at one of the big-box chains? NO…so why would you treat your hearing loss there?*" I don't blame the patient for sometimes entering the office thinking he/she is going to be "sold" something.

My best advice is to steer clear of anybody trying to sell you something. If we go back to Reason #1 above, the patient is likely already nervous because he or she knows the medical diagnosis before ever even stepping foot in the office. Combine that with the fear of "being sold something" and that makes for a pretty nervous patient with his or her guard up.

Unfortunately, much of modern medicine is turning into a commercial advertisement seen on TV that marginalizes the process of treating a medical disorder; and hearing health care is not immune to this. In my office, and the Excellence in Audiology member-clinics across the country, our belief is in the medical evaluation and treatment of hearing loss.

I believe strongly that the proper medical treatment of hearing loss is best left to the clinicians specially trained to understand, diagnose, and treat your hearing loss.

REASON #4 — The Cost.

Actual Cost

We all know somebody, perhaps a family member or a friend, who has spent a significant amount of money on a hearing aid gizmo only to use it as a paperweight or to leave it in his or her sock drawer. And the reason is because the glorified over-priced amplifier that he or she purchased was never truly designed to improve hearing or clarity—it was designed to just make sounds louder. This truly angers me, and while I do believe that the patient plays a significant role in his or her health care decisions and follow-up care, the health care provider also must have a significant responsibility to the patient—even after the patient has left the office.

I have heard many horror stories about patients spending upwards of $10,000 on a pair of hearing aid gizmos—YIKES! More often than not, this very high retail transaction very likely took place in one of the chain hearing aid sales shops (i.e. the "Miracle Hearing" and "Bellstone" shops. FYI the real names of these retail establishments have been altered in an attempt to reduce my chances of being sued!). And, sadly, all the patient got in return for his or her money was a hearing aid amplifier capable of making things louder.

When a practice and the providers are committed to the medical treatment of hearing loss, you can trust that you are in good hands. I believe that a hearing specialist must meet the strict standards required of Excellence in Audiology member-clinics and follow the medical model of treating hearing loss.

I have always believed that the patient needs options to help him or her invest in proper hearing health care. A reputable audiology practice understands that for some people, the upfront investment in hearing healthcare can be prohibitive. Patients must be provided with options. All Excellence In Audiology member-clinics will offer TreatmentFi™, a simple, affordable way to treat hearing loss. This program is subscription-based and provides access to affordable hearing health care without compromise. The TreatmentFi™ program offers a lifetime warranty for all technology (including loss of devices), complete access to supplies and batteries, all treatment and diagnostic appointments, and no-cost automatic upgrades of NeuroTechnology™ as hearing and cognitive needs change.

Hidden Cost

What about the cost of _**not**_ treating hearing loss? While research has yet to make the definitive finding that hearing loss can *cause* dementia (causality is often difficult in clinical science), the evidence that the relationship exists is overwhelming. Even more important is the mounting evidence that treating hearing loss may significantly reduce the risk of developing dementia.

Every day, 10,000 people turn sixty-five years young. This trend is expected to continue for at least the next fifteen years. And it is almost a guarantee that over the next fifteen years, science will continue to reduce the mortality rate and increase the average life expectancy. As a result, our health care system will be pushed to its capacity to deal with diseases such as cancer, diabetes, cardiovascular disease, etc. Perhaps the most prevalent, most costly, and most disabling of all diseases we will see sharply rise over the ensuing decades is dementia—the mind-robbing mental disease that interrupts and interferes with every aspect of life. Dementia is **_not_** a normal part of aging.

Every three to four seconds, another patient is diagnosed with dementia. Rates of dementia are estimated to triple in the next thirty years. Unlike the other diseases listed above, a physical body with dementia is estimated to outlive the individual's mental capabilities by ten or more years! It is estimated that the average cost, per family, to manage the medical treatment and care of a loved one with dementia can exceed $57,000 per year.

There is no cure for this catastrophic disease, but there are treatments available, including several ways to decrease your risk of developing dementia. **In fact, a study published in The Lancet journal indicated that the treatment of hearing loss as the single most effective means of preventing dementia.**

I encourage you to read my report detailing "9 Key Lifestyle Tips to Reduce the Risk of Developing Dementia." This report can be found at *www.ExcellenceInAudiology.org.*

REASON #5 — Everybody *HATES* Hearing Aids.

Let's be honest. Everybody hates hearing aids. In fact, when you make a reference to old-fashioned volume-enhancing hearing aids, I think you could go so far as to say "Some hearing aids suck!" There you have it—I said it! I've been working with hearing-impaired patients for nearly twenty years and although my patients love improved hearing, they hate their hearing aids. I don't see a reason to tip-toe around this subject or ignore the fact that patients generally do not like using hearing aids. Nobody wants a medical disorder that requires physically tethering a device to his or her body to treat the medical condition.

People who wear glasses do not actually *want* to wear glasses (although I do know some people who wear non-prescriptive glasses because they feel that they look "cool"). I remember growing up in a time where people who wore glasses were sometimes referred to as "four-eyes" or other derogatory terms—fortunately glasses are now commonplace for people of all ages. I know that in the next few years, I will likely begin to hold the restaurant menu farther and farther away from my face in a dimly lit restaurant and when that happens I will need to invest in the proper treatment of visual impairment—whether I want to wear glasses or not.

For some people, hearing aids carry the stigma of meaning "I'm old and ready to die." And nearly every day I see a patient try and talk him- or herself out of investing in hearing health care treatment because "eh, I won't be around much longer anyway." My response is always the same: if you live for three more days, three more months, three more years, or even thirty more years (which is not unreasonable to expect from my fifty-eight year young patients), isn't it worth wanting to hear and understand everything and everyone else in your life? I also point out to patients that they will appear to look much older if they continue to say "What?" or "Huh?" all the time or, perhaps even worse, start to isolate themselves from the conversation.

I get it, and I respect that patients don't want to use a hearing aid, whatever the reason may be. Any reputable hearing health care provider will realize this, also, and understand the difference between traditional hearing aids and advanced NeuroTechnology™. Features in NeuroTechnology™ are specifically designed to treat the medical condition of hearing loss, improve cognitive function, and improve overall quality of life. As an added benefit, NeuroTechnology™ is incredibly discrete and comes in several invisible styles (more on invisible hearing-loss treatment options later in the book).

Part 1
Finding a Hearing Health Care Specialist

QUESTION #1

Why is hearing so important?

I believe most people can relate to my story: I watched my grandmother degrade as she crossed over from her seventies to her eighties. As she got older, her hearing got worse—and as the hearing got worse, her cognitive abilities declined. As a result, our ability to communicate with her was significantly strained. This is when I first knew that hearing loss must be correlated to cognitive decline (AKA dementia).

Communication is truly the basic building block of every relationship we have at work, at home with our loved ones, with our children, etc. Communication is a vital part of establishing and maintaining relationships. Watching my grandmother decline helped push me to be a better student, a better teacher, and a better clinician. When I decided to veer from clinical audiology for several years to focus on my studies at M.I.T. and Harvard Medical School, I decided to point my efforts at understanding the neuroscience of how we hear at the most basic level—from vibrating molecules of air to neural activity in the brain. Armed with this knowledge, I have been able to advance my patients' care to the highest level and help to set standards for testing and treatment protocol used in clinics across the country.

QUESTION #2

What are some of the early signs of hearing loss, and when should I see a hearing specialist?

Hearing loss is typically a slow, gradual onset disorder that silently (pardon the pun) affects the individual. The most common symptoms experienced by most (perhaps not all) patients are difficulty hearing in background noise, tinnitus, and thinking most people mumble or speak softly! Most people who experience the initial symptoms of hearing loss do not even realize it is happening. It is far easier to blame the acoustics of the room, the volume of the background noise, or the person speaking (i.e. "they mumble") than it is to accept that it's your hearing that is lacking. It is also difficult for many patients to rationalize the need for medical treatment of hearing loss because in some (ideal listening) situations (i.e. sitting at a table one-on-one in a perfectly quiet environment) may not be much of a challenge. But the truth is...

A Mild Hearing Loss is a Major Problem!

The first symptom of hearing loss for most patients is difficulty hearing in complex listening environments. If you take the time to reflect truly and deeply on your communication breakdown, I believe you will begin to recognize some of the initial symptoms of hearing loss. Are you having any difficulty when there are a few people at the kitchen table? Or when the kids come over? Or when communicating with your grandchildren? Or when you are at a social gathering (i.e. sharing a meal with friends and you can't seem to follow the conversation, yet all the other people seem to be enjoying themselves and following the conversation)? It is in these types of scenarios when hearing loss can really start to rear its ugly head and you realize that you are no longer an active part of the conversation. The result is a slow retraction from contributing to the conversation because you may feel embarrassed, and thus you continue to further isolate yourself and find yourself not truly engaging in conversations and relationships. And this is how even a mild hearing loss can really begin to impact your quality of life and relationships with others.

In addition to the importance of maintaining an active, engaged life with family and friends, early treatment of mild hearing loss is important for maintaining proper brain health. Simply put: Hearing Care is Health Care™. Your hearing drives your conception of everything and everybody around you; thus, hearing is essentially driving cognition at all times. It's driving memory. It's driving your image of the environment around you. You don't turn hearing on or off; you can't close your ears like you can close your eyes. There really isn't a sense or portion of your brain that isn't connected to your auditory system.

And I believe this speaks to how important hearing is to live and to thrive. We are bombarded with sound at all times and the brain is constantly, in real-time, making decisions as to whether or not certain sounds are important, trying to figure out how to categorize the sound and if it is important to store away and remember it for reference at a later date. A mild hearing loss can take away significant portions of the auditory world around you—and is likely the reason behind why patients with untreated hearing loss are at a significantly higher risk of experiencing a devastating fall.

The lack of cognitive stimulation that accompanies even a mild hearing loss is also associated with cognitive decline and dementia. Reports from Johns Hopkins Medical Center (and others) indicate that a <u>mild</u> hearing loss can increase the risk of developing dementia by 200% (up to a 500% increase for those with a severe hearing loss).

Like every major medical condition, the key to successful management of the disorder is early intervention. ***"Catch it early and treat it early!"***

QUESTION #3

Why, and how, should I choose a specialist for my hearing loss treatment?

I get this question so often that I developed a Top 10 List (although it's not nearly as fun as David Letterman's Top 10 Lists). This list can help a patient understand "why" they need to choose a specialist and "how" to choose the right specialist to trust with the treatment of their hearing loss. For a more detailed report than what is provided here, visit *www.ExcellenceInAudiology.org* for the full report.

The Top 10 Things You Must Know before Choosing Your Hearing Health Care Provider

❶ Is He or She a Specialist?

Hearing health care consists of both Audiologist and Hearing Instrument Specialist; both working towards the same goal—to help more people struggling with hearing loss. Audiologists are clinically trained hearing health care specialists that take on several extra years of training in order to provide the most thorough diagnostic evaluation and complete the most comprehensive treatment plans aimed at restoring hearing clarity. Hearing Instrument Specialist are trained and licensed professionals that dispense hearing aids. These hearing health care providers perform auditory rehabilitation, which is likely to include the use of NeuroTechnology™ that provides proper stimulation to the auditory system. This is a fancy way to describe how we normalize the way our brains process the incoming sounds in order to achieve maximum clarity, especially in background noise. While there are many hearing health care providers, less than 2% of all audiologists are Excellence in Audiology members.

As the leader of the Excellence In Audiology movement, I don't just treat hearing problems; I also teach clinicians across the country how to become better hearing health care providers. In fact, I have shared my knowledge and taught hundreds of hearing health care specialists throughout the world. By teaching and interacting with many clinicians, I am able to stay at the cutting edge with the best treatment options for my patients.

Another sign of a great specialist is he or she can show you a before and after of a similar case that he or she has previously helped. We know all ears are different, but with the 100,000+ ears our member-clinics have restored clarity to, we can show you a similar case to your specific hearing situation.

❷ Does the Hearing Health Care Provider Have a Medical Office (or a Sales Office)?

In the audiology world, it is not hard to open up shop on a shoe-string budget and call yourself a specialist. When you are searching for a provider, make sure you understand the clinician's credentials and medical affiliations. Often times, smaller offices with limited staff and audiology providers are somewhat limited in their service offerings and stability.

If you find a hearing care provider with the best credentials and an office that is inviting and in a medical setting, you have found a specialist who understands the importance of hearing health care and will be around for years to come to help you and your family best understand and address your hearing needs. For a list of Excellence In Audiology member-clinics, visit *www.ExcellenceInAudiology.org.*

Excellence in Audiology member-clinics are located across the country with hearing health care clinicians of the highest caliber who insist on the best practice (often setting the standards for best practices) for their patients and loved ones.

❸ Does the Specialist Think Brain First?

Everybody thinks "we hear with our ears," and while that is partially correct, the process of hearing actually happens at the level of the brain. Today's hearing loss treatments are far more than a simple "amplifying" device behind your ear. The neuroscience behind modern treatments is focused on the brain, cognition, and the comorbidities of untreated hearing loss (comorbidity is defined as a disorder that co-occurs/is correlated to hearing loss). If your clinician thinks hearing first and *not* brain first in his or her treatment plan, you are missing out on many long-term lifestyle benefits. NeuroTechnology™ is aimed at restoring lost clarity, providing noise-canceling filters for noisy background situations, and soft-speech enhancers that emphasize the speech of those soft-speakers in your life.

When searching for your hearing health care provider, make sure you find a specialist that understands the significant negative impacts of untreated hearing loss on your brain. To find a local clinician who has been recognized for their commitment to thinking brain first in treatment plans, prescriptions, and protocols, you can visit the website *www.ExcellenceInAudiology.org.*

❹ Do They Include a Free Consultation at the Initial Appointment?

Most audiologists and hearing specialists offer free consultations for new patients so that you and your family can get expert advice about treatment needs, options, and timing before making this important investment.

During your first evaluation and consultation, be sure your questions are being answered, your concerns are being addressed, and you are being educated about all of your treatment options. The clinician should include a comprehensive written report during, or after, the evaluation at no charge.

❺ Does the Specialist's Office Offer Guarantees? If So, What Are They?

No matter which hearing health care provider you choose, ultimately you are not making a small investment—in both time and finances. That being said, it is important to know that your clinician is going to stand behind his or her medical treatment plan. Every Excellence in Audiology member-clinic offers multiple guarantees.

In addition to a 100% Money-Back Clarity Guarantee, be sure your specialist offers a lifetime guarantee on service and prescription programming.

Rest assured—your hearing health care is my priority. Thus, I stand by everything I've recommended in this publication and why I have chosen to lead the Excellence in Audiology movement.

❻ Is He or She Using the Latest Technology and Treatment Options Available?

Audiology today differs a great deal from years past. Computer-designed NeuroTechnology™ devices and wireless technologies dramatically increase the precision with which we restore clarity and boost hearing ability. Scientific verification of device settings, while in your ear (referred to as Real Ear Measurements) maximize the precision of NeuroTechnology™ benefits. As an added incentive, today's NeuroTechnology™ are discrete and virtually undetectable to the user and others. In fact, a new category of NeuroTechnology™, known for being invisible, can offer the most discrete, cosmetically pleasing option placed deep in your ear canal to make the entire treatment a well-kept secret!

❼ Does Your Investment Include Treatment Supplies?

Each hearing care office has its own fee schedules, and specialists often charge differently for procedures. All specialists should offer you a contract which clearly spells out the investment for you or your loved one's treatment before it begins.

❽ Does the Specialist Charge for Follow-Up and Emergency Appointments?

Each time a patient embarks on the journey of improved hearing, there is an adaptation period for the user's ears and brain to adjust. This period can take thirty to forty-five days and is individual to each patient. In addition to the complex cognitive changes that happen when restoring hearing clarity, patients will notice significant improvement in some hearing situations and perhaps not as much in some other situations. This is common in the initial process of hearing loss treatments. I believe every patient is entitled to complimentary customizations for their NeuroTechnology™ prescription.

Keep in mind, if your NeuroTechnology™ is broken or damaged due to non-compliance with care, protection, and maintenance, this may result in repair charges. As a simple rule, if you do your best to avoid breaking your NeuroTechnology™ and follow the simple guidelines that your audiology specialist shares with you, then you should have no additional costs for customizations, even if it's an "emergency."

❾ Does the Clinician Make You Feel Special and Comfortable?

When you meet with your hearing health care provider, the person you are trusting with your hearing health care, you need to be in a comfortable and welcoming environment. Each Excellence in Audiology member-clinic I work with understands the importance of hearing and the distress that can be involved with making the decision to treat one's hearing loss. The entire experience from beginning to end, including a welcoming staff, should be designed to help alleviate a person's feeling of anxiety or grief.

We believe every patient is special and must be made to feel that way every time he or she comes to one of our offices in need of hearing health care.

❿ Does the Specialist Have a Great Reputation?

With the internet today, it is extremely easy to pull up ratings and reviews from patients. Simply go to Google and search for audiology reviews and ratings within your town. At the time of this report, my practice in Worcester, Massachusetts, and our Intermountain Audiology clinics in the west, along with Excellence in Audiology member-clinics across the country have amassed thousands of five-star reviews on Google, Facebook, and HealthyHearing.com. No other network even comes close to this number of reviews. In fact, most of our offices have other providers in their area that have either no ratings or many poor ratings.

And don't be shy about asking for references—go directly to the source! You have the right to call any audiology office and ask for a list of references, including other patients and local physicians that have volunteered to help advise patients as they first enter the (sometimes overwhelming) world of hearing loss and to help patients understand rehabilitation experiences from the first-person perspective.

QUESTION #4

How early in life should I have my hearing evaluated?

The Simple Answer

If you are over fifty, you should have your hearing evaluated.

Detailed Answer

I have tried to stress the importance of early diagnosis and treatment of hearing loss throughout this book and to each of my patients.

The American Speech Language Hearing Association, the American Academy of Audiology, and the American Medical Association have all considered the recommendation of including "hearing evaluation/screening" between the ages of fifty to sixty years young. I often use the catch phrase "Ears and Rears" as my way of getting people to remember to have their hearing checked when they turn fifty (and of course, have a colon cancer screening too!).

Similar to going to your primary care physician every year, obtaining a baseline hearing test can help to better serve you and your clinician as a guide to the medical recommendation at current or future appointments. Obtaining a baseline evaluation and discovering that you have normal hearing never hurt anyone!

Regardless of age, if you are noticing any of the symptoms of hearing loss (e.g. difficulty hearing in noisy situations, difficulty hearing the TV compared to others), if your family is suggesting you get a hearing test, or if you have ringing in your ears (defined as tinnitus), then it is time to take the first step and have your hearing evaluated and discuss treatment options.

Unfortunately, waiting too long can significantly impact the expectations and outcome of treatment, and sadly every hearing health care clinician I know has a patient they have had to tell he or she waited too long and the benefits of treatment will be minimal.

Part 2
Fixing the Right Things at the Right Time

QUESTION #5

What will happen at the initial evaluation and consultation?

Every process has a beginning, middle, and end.

The Beginning

First things first…your specialist will ask you "Why are you here today?" (or some variation of that "why" question). This helps to set the stage for understanding your specific hearing related issues, concerns, and experiences. This conversation is the baseline to helping your specialist understand why you "raised your hand and are seeking help." While my job title may be "audiologist," this initial line of questioning is designed to help me better understand my patient at a deeper, more emotional level. I want to know my patient's experience with hearing loss and how it impacts his/her life. How does your hearing loss impact your relationship with your grandchildren? How does hearing loss impact your relationship with your spouse? Does hearing loss get in the way of your performance at work? Some of my patients wait their entire life to go fishing with their grandchild, and now their hearing loss is robbing them of the richness of that experience and getting in the way of developing a deeper relationship. As an audiologist, it is my job to treat ***your*** hearing loss and ***you*** as a person.

The Middle

Treating hearing loss is a process steeped in science, engineering, technology, and clinical medicine. There is also an "art" to treating hearing loss, and this skill is developed with years of experience. In order to develop the right treatment plan for each patient, first there must be the proper diagnostic procedures that test every aspect of hearing.

First your clinician will observe the ear canal to make sure the canals are free of any obstructing cerumen (ear wax). This is most often followed by a procedure called tympanometry that can rule out any medical condition causing hearing loss involving the eardrum and/or the space behind it, including the middle ear bones (the "Hammer, Anvil, and Stirrup").

The Beeps!

From there, it is important to establish the degree of hearing loss (ranked from mild to profound). Using the "raise your hand when you hear the beep" may conjure memories of having your hearing screened by the school nurse, but it still serves a purpose: establishing the degree of hearing loss. If your specialist stops testing you at that point and makes a recommendation for treating your hearing loss…I advise you to run as fast as you can! The information gathered from this test, although important, is only a piece of the puzzle.

The Words!

The most important testing we will perform is designed to assess your cognitive hearing, e.g. how well do you understand words in quiet and with background noise (after all, nobody comes to the office complaining that they can't hear beeps!). This line of testing will truly help your clinician understand how well you hear, and how well you process words and conversation.

Testing a patient's ability to hear words is often referred to as "Word Discrimination Scores/Ability." First the patient is asked to repeat a list of words at a near-normal conversational volume. Individuals with normal hearing will always correctly repeat between 96-100% of the words on this test. Individuals with hearing loss will not score nearly as well. For example, many people with a mild to moderate hearing age-related hearing loss will typically score between 50-60%—thus the patient is expected to miss 40-50% of what is said to him or her on a daily basis (especially when visual and contextual cues are removed and only hearing is utilized).

The next test is a repeat, almost exactly as just described, but performed a second time at a volume and clarity setting ideal for the specific patient's hearing loss. The result of this second round of word testing is referred to as the patient's "Hearing Potential Score." Most often the patient who formerly scored between 50-60% will now score 90% and greater; thus, treatment with NeuroTechnology™ is expected to improve the patient's hearing clarity to 90% and greater on a daily basis (especially in a quiet conversational setting). The patient is fully aware that he or she performed significantly better with enhanced clarity.

I mentioned earlier that the consequences of waiting too long to treat hearing loss can be dire. In some cases when the second round of word testing is completed, the patient's "Hearing Potential Score" will sometimes only be as high as 50-60%. In these cases, the outcomes and expectations for treatment are very dim (especially when compared with the patient who scored over 90%).

The Words In Background Noise!

The #1 complaint of every patient with hearing loss, and most often the first symptom of hearing loss, is difficulty understanding speech and conversation in background noise. Thus, it is critical that the clinician understands each patient's ability to decipher speech in background noise (again, without visual or contextual cues). This test, called the Quick Speech in Noise Test (QuickSIN™), is a means to quantify a patient's difficulty understanding and following speech in background noise.

Briefly, the sentence intended to be heard and repeated by the listener is presented at a clear and audible volume to the patient. With each new sentence introduced, the level of background noise (often referred to as "cocktail party noise") is increased in increments of five decibels. The final iteration of the test is when the speech and background "babble" are presented at the same volume—significantly taxing the auditory system and its noise-reduction filters.

Individuals with normal hearing are typically capable of hearing every word at each level, and even most of the words at the final, most competitive level. In contrast, individuals with even a mild hearing loss can struggle significantly on this test when the noise is ten decibels less than the intended speech. The test is scored on a Hearing Handicap Scale and can range from normal, to mild, to moderate, to severe Hearing Handicap. A majority of patients with a mild age-related hearing loss will often score in the mild to moderate hearing handicap range, confirming his or her reported difficulty following conversation in complex listening situations.

The End

Once all the testing is complete, it is the clinician's responsibility to review all test results with the patient and with his or her loved ones. These results are personal and can help a patient better understand the difficulty he or she is dealing with on a daily basis. Understanding the results can also be just as important for family and loved ones.

Although an individual with normal hearing can only imagine what it feels like to suffer from permanent hearing loss, gaining an understanding of the degree of hearing loss, Hearing Potential Ability, and Hearing Handicap scores can help the loved ones gain perspective on what the patient is going through and how much of a strain hearing loss can be.

These test results will determine the medical treatment plan and help initiate the journey towards improved hearing clarity and cognitive health.

QUESTION #6

What if I still have questions after the initial consultation?

The initial consultation can be overwhelming for some people and for their family members—and can sometimes stretch to sixty minutes or more. In these situations, it can be difficult to ask every question, to process everything that is being said, and to understand the enormity of the diagnosis of hearing loss. Every patient of mine has my e-mail, office phone number, and I've even gone so far as to include my cell phone number on my business card. I believe in an open discussion and dialogue and that many patients, and perhaps their family members, will have questions that come up even after the appointment is over.

I always invite and encourage patients to bring family and loved ones to their appointments. Bring a spouse, bring a child, bring a grandchild—it's okay because your hearing loss impacts every one of these people.

It is important that the patient and his or her loved ones understand exactly what is happening with the patient, exactly what the degree of hearing loss is, how the disorder can impact his or her life, how it can impact his or her cognitive function, and how it can impact his or her risk of developing dementia, which often leads to loss of independence and even institutionalization. At the initial consultation, there will also be a medical recommendation presented for how to treat the hearing loss. There is no one-size-fits-all treatment plan. NeuroTechnology™ offers a wide array of options that are often dictated by the test results and patients' needs.

QUESTION #7

When is the best time to treat my hearing loss?

A.S.A.P. Hearing loss is associated with increased rates of diabetes, heart disease, kidney disease, thyroid disease, falling, and the development of dementia.

The longer you wait, the more you are depriving the brain of proper auditory stimulation, often referred to as *auditory deprivation*. Your brain is not getting the proper auditory stimulation and auditory cues that it needs to run at 100%. The brain is a very simple "Use it or Lose It" mechanism, and auditory input can help to provide the proper, constant stimulation our brains are accustomed to and designed to receive.

Hearing is not a sense to take for granted. Yet the statistics are alarming—it is estimated that only 20% of individuals with hearing loss actually seek medical treatment. Without the proper treatment of hearing loss, the brain is being asked to work on overload, constantly. I often use the analogy "living with untreated hearing loss is like asking your brain to drive sixty miles per hour in second gear."

In neuroscience, we call this "Cognitive Overload"—asking the brain to process auditory, visual, and other cues just to put together a simple sentence.

Consider this sentence:

> *Hi, Martha! How is your puppy doing? Is he eating and growing*
> *OK? I hope we can get our dogs together soon to play.*

If we filter this sentence through a typical mild age-related hearing loss with compromised clarity (e.g. difficulty with consonant discrimination), the sentence could be perceived as this:

> *i, Mara! ow i our uy oing? I e eaing and groing o? I oe e an ge our*
> *do ogeer oon o ay.*

I think you will agree that this is rather alarming. Remember earlier when we discussed patients with mild hearing loss missing 50-60% of words at near-normal conversational volume? This is what it could sound like to the patient with auditory-only cues. Of course, the brain will use visual cues, lip-reading, etc. to fill in the missing pieces—but the brain was not designed to take on that much stress and effort just to understand a simple sentence.

This cognitive overload is hypothesized to be one of the leading reasons that individuals with hearing loss can be ***FIVE TIMES*** more likely to develop dementia.

QUESTION #8

What if I am nervous about treating my hearing loss?

Undergoing treatment for any medical disorder can be overwhelming to patients and to their family members. Fortunately, today's NeuroTechnology™ has alleviated most of the worries and concerns about treating hearing loss. The technology is specifically designed to be discretely worn all day and fit comfortably in the patient's ear. With enhanced clarity features, background noise cancellation filters, and wireless connectivity, today's hearing loss treatment options are simple and sometimes even fun—you can connect your NeuroTechnology™ to all sorts of home electronics including light bulbs, coffee pots, door bells, etc.—but this is beyond the scope of this book!

QUESTION #9

Why can't we wait until next year to treat my hearing loss?

Hearing loss, for some reason, seems to be the perfect thing for patients to try and put off "until next year." Patients will try to rationalize their hearing loss: "Oh, this is normal for my age" or "Everybody mumbles." If patients don't understand the unintended consequences of waiting to treat hearing loss and the medical conditions associated with hearing loss, how can they be expected to understand the importance of starting treatment of hearing loss **today!**

Simply stated, the organ of hearing (i.e. the cochlea) has a finite amount of receptor cells—referred to as hair cells. The hair cells are akin to the rods and cones of the eye, which receive stimulation and pass along the information as a complex series of neurochemical signals to the brain. As we age, like most mammals roaming the planet, humans are genetically predetermined to suffer the effects of age-related hearing loss. This problem is becoming more prominent in our society as we live longer, more active and engaged lives.

With this progressive degenerative disorder, there is a gradual, continual loss of hair cells within the cochlea. These cells each have upwards of thirty nerve fibers responsible for relaying information to the brain to process sounds and conversation. As each cell dies with age and excessive exposure to noise (compounded by the combination of the two), the cells will die and so, too, will the attached neurons.

A recent study from Johns Hopkins found significant cerebral atrophy (AKA brain shrinkage) in the brains of individuals with hearing loss—likely the result of the progressive degenerative nature of hearing loss. The cerebral atrophy found in these individuals is reminiscent of the global cerebral atrophy observed in individuals with dementia.

Treating hearing loss early has many advantages—predicated on "Use It or (Continue to) Lose It." Treating hearing loss cannot prevent further damage caused by our genetics or prior exposure to loud noise, but it can help maintain clarity and fine resolution of speech understanding as the disorder progresses. For example, a study I worked on at Brooklyn College (CUNY) graduate school under the supervision of Dr. Shlomo Silman was attempting to understand the impact of only using one hearing aid when the patient had equal amounts of hearing loss in both ears. The results were pretty alarming.

The untreated ear's ability to perform word discrimination tasks significantly reduced compared to the treated ear. Looking back on these results, they almost seem like common sense—the brain was designed to receive input from two ears and can respond adversely if only stimulated by one. I often joke with my patients who ask, "Do I have to treat both ears?" by asking them "How many *Monopoly-men* do you know walking around with a monocle!" In all seriousness, the importance of treating hearing loss early cannot be understated. Maintaining the strength and vitality of neural connections of the ear to the brain is key to the successful treatment of hearing loss.

Part 3
Focusing on a Plan That Works for You

Is there an ideal patient?

The ideal patient is a person who understands both the medical and personal consequences of untreated hearing loss. A person who understands that his/her hearing loss is not just about him/her, but that hearing loss impacts his/her entire family, group of friends, and community. An ideal patient is somebody who is invested in his/her life, somebody who is invested in active aging, somebody who is invested in living independently, somebody who wants to stay engaged and who wants to be a part of the conversation, somebody who wants to be a part of his/her family and who wants to be a part of their community.

The ideal patient has to accept the cost-benefit ratio when it comes to treating hearing loss; and I hope that this book has helped patients understand that it's nearly impossible to put a dollar value on improved health. I believe the ideal patient truly wants to stay involved, wants to grow, wants to remain independent, and wants to make the most of every day and every relationship that he or she has. That is an ideal patient. If you are, or know someone that fits this description, please help them begin treatment of their hearing loss as soon as possible. You are always welcome at my center or at one of the Excellence in Audiology member-clinics in your area.

I suppose on the other side of the coin is the "not ideal patient"—the person who has his wife, his kids, and his grandkids basically pushing him into the office. That's not an ideal patient, although we have helped motivate many of them to realize what they need to do for themselves and their families. This type of patient must realize the severity of their situation and they must want to make a change. As you know, "you can lead a horse to water, but you can't make it drink."

QUESTION #10

What treatment options are available to me when I'm ready to start treating my hearing loss?

I get this question often as I travel the country meeting new patients, and even from family and friends. My answer is always the same: **NeuroTechnology**™. Advances in technology specifically designed to treat the cognitive aspects of hearing loss, not just make things louder, have significantly improved patient care and patient satisfaction.

But, my next response is always *"You must see an Excellence in Audiology member-clinic to determine which form of NeuroTechnology*™ *suits you and your hearing loss best."*

While the most important factor in determining treatment is always based on the patient's hearing profile and health care history, specific options can be based on several factors including: addressing specific patient symptoms (difficulty in certain acoustic environments, tinnitus, etc.), dexterity (can the patient manipulate an invisible hearing device?), and personal preferences (color, size, etc.,). Your hearing health care provider can help you understand which form of NeuroTechnology™, what shape and size, and which specific features can help you hear your best and keep you engaged in conversation.

QUESTION #11

What treatment options are available for the ringing in my ears (aka tinnitus)?

As a Neuroscientist and Clinical Audiologist, one of the most common questions, **and complaints**, I get from my patients is about the 'ringing' in their ears! Tinnitus (pronounced either TIH·nih·tus or tuh·NYE·tus) is defined as a sensation of sound in your ears, sometimes in your head. Each person with tinnitus has a different sound experience; for most it is described as a "ringing" sound, but many patients also report a shooshing, buzzing, or wooshing sound—similar to the sounds inside a conch shell.

It is currently estimated that nearly 50,000,000 American adults live with tinnitus. Tinnitus is experienced by approximately 80% of people living with hearing loss.

Too many people dismiss the ringing, when in fact this sound essentially represents an internal alarm alerting you that something is not as it should be. Whether the tinnitus is constant, only noticeable in a quiet room or at night, pulsating or seems to have certain triggers (i.e. exercise or caffeine), it is important that the root cause of the problem be determined and a proper treatment plan be put in place with your hearing health care specialist. In some people, the tinnitus can interfere with daily life and result in depression, anxiety and affect concentration.

What is the cause of tinnitus?

The most common cause of tinnitus is damage to the sensory organ of hearing, the cochlea (i.e. the inner ear). The cochlea is to hearing what your eyes are to vision. Within the cochlea are tiny hair-like cells, called hair cells. When these cells are damaged, the nerves that connect the hair cells to the brain (and give us the ability to hear), become permanently damaged; and often times the ringing will ensue.

How Do the Sensory Cells In My Ear Get Damaged?

The sensory cells in the ear are most vulnerable to aging. Think about it—as we get older, we tend not to see as well or see as sharply as we used to, especially in low-light environments. Unfortunately, the same process happens in our ears as we age; we tend not to hear as clearly, especially in noisy situations.

Another common cause of tinnitus is excessive noise exposure, either a single intense noise (like a shotgun blast) or long-term exposure either from work or play (e.g. musicians, concert attendees, carpenters, machinist, landscapers, etc.).

But Why Do My Ears Ring?

Tinnitus is most often the result of a "Central Gain" in neural activity that occurs when there is a loss of proper neural stimulation from the ear to the brain. More simply, when the brain is not properly stimulated in individuals with hearing loss (even a mild hearing loss), the brain will increase activity to make up for the missing input.

This "Central Gain" is neurologically analogous to "Phantom Limb" phenomenon studied in neuroscience. In cases where damage occurs to the peripheral nervous system—such as when a solider loses a limb in battle—the central nervous system (aka the brain) will undergo adaptive changes that can often result in the perception of pain. Our ear's perception of pain is the ringing.

Treatment For Your Tinnitus

Unfortunately, too many patients have said to me, "I have tinnitus, and I've been told there is nothing that I can do about it." I emphatically say to each of these patients—that is not true! Is there a cure for tinnitus? No. Are there proven FDA-approved treatment options available to reduce, and in some cases, eliminate, the ringing? YES!

The single most effective treatment option available for patients suffering with tinnitus is NeuroTechnology™. The FDA (Food and Drug Administration) has approved treatment for individuals with tinnitus by providing the brain with restored proper stimulation. And while most people with tinnitus also suffer with hearing loss, that is not always the case. Fortunately, newly available NeuroTechnology™ has been designed for people with hearing loss and for individuals with (so called) "normal" hearing. Many studies show that patients who use the tinnitus support technology note a significant reduction in their daily tinnitus experience—with some even reporting that "the ringing is gone all day."

QUESTION #12

What if I have "total hearing loss" in one of my ears? (And what is a CROS System?)

As a general rule of thumb, hearing ability in the two ears should be near equal to each other. After all, your ears are the same age. If you have a history of noise exposure it was likely the same in both ears, and if you were prescribed a medicine with a side-effect that could impact hearing, it would impact both ears similarly.

But, in some patients, hearing in one ear will diverge from the other. This can result from a host of otologic issues, including viral infection of the ear, physical trauma to the ear, and of unknown origin (medically diagnosed as "idiopathic hearing loss," which is my favorite medical diagnosis because the root meaning of the phrase "idiopathic" is that the clinicians are idiots and don't know what happened! Ha! I don't say that to disparage any clinicians—it's just sometimes we can't figure out why the patient has worse hearing in one ear).

The separation of hearing levels between the two ears can sometimes be dramatic or even complete. Unfortunately, some patients have a "dead ear" (medically defined as anacusis) with normal hearing in the other ear. In other patients, there is an "asymmetric hearing loss" which implies hearing loss in one ear and even worse hearing in the other ear.

The brain was designed to hear with two ears, and it will function best with equal hearing in both ears. Binaural (two-ear) hearing has significant benefits that include increased sound localization ability (e.g. figuring out where sound is coming from in the room) and enhanced perception of speech in noisy situations. These characteristics of binaural hearing are often referred to as the "Binaural Advantage." If you know somebody with "lopsided" hearing loss, you will notice that she always strategizes to improve the listening environment by having the speaker(s) on her better hearing side.

While the course of treatment for individuals with significantly poorer hearing in one ear is different than the patient with symmetrical hearing loss, NeuroTechnology™ can be used to significantly enhance hearing and understanding in all listening situations.

Briefly, the most common NeuroTechnology™ used in these cases is referred to as a CROS System. CROS (Contralateral Routing of Signal) will take sound from the "dead" / worse side and route it over to the better side (even if there is some hearing loss in the "better" side). Using this technology allows the patient to access sound on the (otherwise) muted side of the body. While this patient may never perform as well as an individual treating equal levels of hearing loss in both ears, restoring perception of sound from the muted side of the body can offer significant relief in almost all listening situations.

QUESTION #13

Do they still make traditional hearing aids?

Yes, traditional hearing aids are still made. Mostly this traditional technology has been relabeled and is now masquerading as "new" over-the-counter (OTC) technology or personal sound amplification devices (PSAPs). Unfortunately, because the words "hearing aid" are very general and very common, it can be quite confusing for the patient. As I explain to my patients nearly every day:

"Your father (or grandfather) wore traditional hearing aids (and he probably hated them). This older technology was intended to make sounds louder regardless of location in the room, regardless of the volume of the incoming sounds, and regardless of what the patient did or didn't actually want to hear."

As an audiologist seeing patients early on in my career, I was very disappointed by the limitations of the traditional hearing aid technology (and often embarrassed about having to relay the cost of the device—knowing the benefit would be limited, thereby limiting the patient's ability to remain socially engaged). This high level of patient dissatisfaction played a role in my decision to "take a break" from clinical audiology for nearly six years and pursue my studies in neuroscience.

QUESTION #14

So, what's the deal with new hearing aids and Neuro Technology™?

(Most) new "hearing aids" are NeuroTechnology™.

To continue my answer from the last question: when I decided to come back to audiology as a clinical fellow at the Brigham and Women's Hospital in Boston and then as clinical professor at Northeastern University, I was instantly relieved at the giant leaps and bounds hearing aids had made towards improving listening experience for the patient (and thus increasing patient satisfaction). Around this time, the average patient satisfaction rating for traditional hearing aid experience was hovering around 70% to 75% (as measured by the MarkeTrak survey).

If you now fast-forward another ten years to present time, the most recent MarkeTrack survey examining patient satisfaction with hearing loss treatment has shown an **improvement to 91%!** I believe this number speaks for itself.

Treatment of hearing loss with traditional hearing aids is (thankfully) beginning to be phased out and replaced with NeuroTechnology™ designed to enhance hearing in all listening situations, enhance clarity of speech details, automatically provide an increased boost of volume for soft speakers, stimulate the brain, and increase cognitive function.

QUESTION #15

What in the heck is an invisible hearing aid?

I saved my favorite treatment topic for last...*invisible hearing aids*. Like Wonder Woman's invisible jet plane—you can't see it, but it kicks butt! I get questions about this all the time from patients: "What is an invisible hearing aid?" and "Will my friends be able to see it?"

When treating hearing loss with NeuroTechnology™, I have two principles that I always follow:

1. Use the right NeuroTechnology™ to treat the patient's hearing loss and improve cognitive health.

2. Respect the patient's desire for NeuroTechnology™ that is physically and aesthetically comfortable for them.

BUT... Principle #2 can _never_ override Principle #1.

As a general rule of thumb in the tech world, the size of technology decreases over time. NeuroTechnology™ uses smaller, more powerful digital technology and processing to automatically adapt to the user's surroundings. I have always believed that treating hearing loss should require minimal effort from the patient. The hearing-impaired person needs to start using NeuroTechnology™ when he or she wakes up in the morning and then simply remove it before falling asleep—and do *nothing* in between! NeuroTechnology™ has ushered in the age of *effortless* hearing loss treatment.

Advances in design and technology allow for the user to be hands free—no more buttons for environment (i.e. push the button twice when in a noisy restaurant, push three times when in the gym, push the button four times when on the phone, etc.) and no more spin-wheels to adjust the volume up and down. Innovations in NeuroTechnology™ allow for automatic adaptation to dynamic environmental listening situations (e.g. listening to speech as you go from a quiet room to a noisy room), and it can automatically adapt to incoming volume to maintain the normal fluctuations in the volume of voices and background noise. The most advanced feature of NeuroTechnology™ is noise-cancellation that delivers increased access to <u>clear</u> speech in noisy listening situations (more on this in the bonus question!).

While NeuroTechnology™ is the circuitry inside the device, the device can come in different shapes and sizes to best fit your hearing loss and your ear.

NeuroTechnology™ Options for Treating Hearing Loss

Invisible Treatment Options

Once placed in your ear, this technology is hassle-free—you may even forget you're wearing the device! And that's the point. Hearing loss shouldn't hold you back, and neither should your hearing solution. Features in today's invisible technology options include:

- An invisible and custom fit
- A deep fit inside your ear canal and personal customization to you for all-day comfort
- Easy adaptation to new sounds with automatic volume control and adaptation to the listening environment
- Wireless streaming to your smartphone to keep you connected to your TV, music, and other media
- Sound comfort technology designed to provide distortion-free listening comfort for loud sounds while ensuring ultimate clarity

*Invisible technology is seated comfortably in the ear canal
for all day comfort and maximum discreteness.*

Mini "Receiver in the Ear" Options

Groundbreaking NeuroTechnology™ is fast and precise enough to analyze and follow the dynamics of the entire auditory environment and differentiate between speech and background noise. Briefly (and without getting too lost in technical details), NeuroTechnology™ is capable of sampling sounds in the environment 100 times per second to make a decision on how to optimally perform and restore clarity; whereas traditional hearing aids were barely capable of analyzing the sound environment and capped out at a sampling rate of less that five times per second.

Advances in miniaturization of technology have led to the breakthrough of new NeuroTechnology™ found to support brain function, including working memory, selective attention, and processing speed (see Bibliography section for report from Dr.

Desjardin, University of Texas, El Paso). These new devices have three features designed specifically to maintain the brain's innate ability to hear in all different listening situations:

- **Clear Hearing in Background Noise.** By separating important speech from background noise by as much as 10 decibels, this new technology provides 30% better speech understanding and clarity in noise*.

- **Enhanced Clarity = Enhanced Memory Recall.** Individuals with hearing loss can have difficulty with working memory, thought to be the result of distorted auditory input to the brain. NeuroTechnology™ can provide 20% more capacity to recall and remember words* by increasing the clarity of the signal being processed by the brain.

- **Reduced Mental Effort.** Many patients describe hearing loss as being "exhausting." Normal hearing is relatively effortless in most listening situations. But to an individual with hearing loss, even a simple conversation at work with a colleague or while out fishing with the grandchildren can require significant effort and use of all available mental resources, including lip-reading. NeuroTechnology™ can offer the hearing-impaired user relief by reducing the "cognitive load" (e.g. mental effort) by 20%*; making the conversation significantly easier to follow in all situations.

Compared to traditional hearing aids

Other features include:

- Hands-free wireless surround sound hearing on the phone.

- Low-battery reminders. Devices can remind you by ear, phone, text, or email that your batteries (or your spouse's batteries) are low.

- Wireless compatibility with any TV to enhance the clarity of the signal.

- Control of your internet connected devices at home, including the thermostat, lights, and even certain cooking appliances.

Let's join in with all current NeuroTechnology™ users and celebrate!

Gone are the days of clunky "beige banana" hearing aids!

Part 4

Financing Your Hearing Loss Treatment without Breaking the Bank

QUESTION #16

How much will my "new ears" cost me?

Answer: It depends.

Throughout this book I have alluded to NeuroTechnology™ treatment options as the "gold standard" of treating hearing loss. Specific recommendations will rely on a number of factors (e.g. degree of hearing loss, symptoms, amount of time living with untreated hearing loss, etc.). However, with that said, I have over twenty years of horror stories of patients trying to "*save a buck.*" I know patients who have thrown away $30, $300, even as much as $3,000 on a "sound machine in their ear" that amplifies volume. Some have tried traditional hearing aids that only make sounds louder; some have tried over-the-counter (OTC) devices; some have tried Personal Sound Amplifiers (PSAPs); some have even tried "mail-order" hearing aids. Regardless, each time the patient comes in professing his *mea culpa* and seeking forgiveness. I take no issue with patients trying to save money and make good economic decisions, but even with health care…you get what you pay for.

Treating the progressive degenerative nature of age-related hearing loss is no different than treating other major medical disorders as you age.

As an example, imagine yourself, or a loved one, in a situation where hip-replacement surgery is required. Could you imagine your surgeon asking the following question?

> "*Would you like me to replace your hip and restore 30%, 70%, or maximum percent mobility?*"

Here is another example, imagine saying to your heart surgeon, after he/she lets you know that you are required to undergo triple by-pass and heart valve replacement:

"Doc, if you don't mind, I'm going to shop on Amazon for a replacement valve to try and save a few bucks...even if it doesn't pump the adequate amount of blood to keep my body oxygenated and healthy."

While both of these scenarios may seem far-fetched and ridiculous, unfortunately the retail aspect of hearing health care has "poisoned the well" for too many people living with hearing loss and has made treating hearing loss a very confusing, onerous process for the patient.

We trust all of our health care providers to use their knowledge and experience to provide us with the best, most medically sound treatment recommendation, ***regardless of price***. You should expect the same from your doctor of audiology. If your clinician is reputable (e.g. is referred to by local physicians, has many five-star reviews on Google, has readily available current patient liaisons to speak with, etc.), is an Excellence in Audiology member-clinic, and has longevity in the community, then you can rest assured that their pricing structure is standard and that the only variable is the cost of technology (pre-set by the technology manufacturer).

NeuroTechnology™ is the #1 most effective, FDA (Food and Drug Administration) approved treatment for hearing loss and has the highest recorded level of patient satisfaction.

QUESTION #17

What is the cost of <u>not</u> treating my hearing loss?

Answer: Possibly a lot more than you think!

Throughout this book we have discussed the positive impact of treating hearing loss and the dire consequences of not treating hearing loss. It is difficult to assign a true monetary value to both of these scenarios, but I will give it my best shot!

Here are two examples.

1. **Hearing loss can increase the risk of developing dementia by 200-500%.** Treating hearing loss is reported as the single most effective modifiable factor to preventing dementia. Given these two medical research findings, it is not unreasonable to calculate the cost of treating a patient with dementia that could have possibly been avoided by treating his or her hearing loss at an earlier age. Statistics show that the average family will spend approximately $57,000 per year to cover health care costs and manage the care of a loved one with dementia.

2. **Hearing loss increases the risk of falls in seniors.** Treating hearing loss can significantly reduce the risk of falling. Again, given these two medical research findings, it is not unreasonable to calculate the cost of treating a patient who falls and compare it to the cost of treating hearing loss. Falling over the age of sixty-five is the #1 cause of injury related deaths. And once a person falls, he or she is two times more likely to fall again. The Center for Disease Control and Prevention (CDC) estimates that the average medical cost associated with a fall that results in hospitalization is over $30,000 (and the cost of treatment increases with age).

In addition to dementia and falls, co-morbidity of hearing loss (i.e. other diseases that are correlated with hearing loss) extends to diabetes, coronary disease, thyroid disease, and others.

QUESTION #18

How do I pay for treatment and what is TreatmentFi™?

"Patients must be provided affordable treatment options when investing in the medical treatment of hearing loss." —Dr. Keith N. Darrow

Like any major medical procedure, the treatment of hearing loss and associated cognitive needs can be expensive, and much of it will *not* covered by your insurance. Unfortunately, price is the most common reason that patients reject the medical treatment of hearing loss. And perhaps an additional problem is that expensive traditional hearing aids never really worked—thus there was little value in paying such a high price. But that has all changed. NeuroTechnology™ is designed to treat the cognitive aspects of hearing loss, and with TreatmentFi™, treatment is now affordable and designed for patients to begin treatment on day one.

For too long I have worked with too many patients who were eager to start treatment of their hearing loss only to be held back by the cost. This motivated me to go back to the drawing board and re-think how we could make hearing health care affordable. I'm so proud that after years of many sleepless nights and way too much time dealing with lawyers and bankers, **we now offer a program that provides access to affordable hearing health care—without compromise.** In the past, if a patient wanted to save a few bucks, they had to even further reduce the effectiveness of traditional hearing aids, but this is no longer an issue for our patients.

TreatmentFi™ has been approved by all 50 state attorney generals for use as an affordable means of treating hearing loss. Each Excellence in Audiology member-clinic offers this new TreatmentFi™ program to their patients. In addition to removing the barrier for my new patients to invest in proper hearing health care, this program also tackles another major issue: patients who have traditional hearing aids but are worried about the cost of upgrading treatment with NeuroTechnology™. This is why I have devised TreatmentFi™ to include no-cost changes to technology every 3 1/2 to 4 years based on changes to the patient's hearing and cognitive needs.

The TreatmentFi™ program at Excellence In Audiology member-clinics is all-inclusive and ensures that each patient always has what is best to treat his or her hearing loss and cognitive needs. With TreatmentFi™, the leader in financing hearing health treatment, our patients have access to low-cost monthly treatment plans that provide significant benefits, including full warranty coverage on treatment technology (including loss, damage, and repair coverage for life); complete access to supplies, batteries, and service appointments; and most importantly, ***no-cost automatic upgrades*** on new treatment technology. The fact of the matter is that not only will a patient's hearing and cognitive needs change over time, but technology will also improve. With TreatmentFi™, treating patients is the top priority!

The benefits of treating your hearing loss with the exclusive TreatmentFi™ process are unlike any other treatment plans available to patients. Each patient that begins treatment of their hearing loss can expect the following benefits:

- A pair of adaptive NeuroTechnology™ is designed to address the cognitive aspects of hearing loss
- Lifetime hearing loss coverage with affordable fixed monthly treatment plan costs
- Lifetime warranty (including a one-time loss)
- Automatic technology upgrades every 48 months (or less)

- Access to discounted technology accessories including rechargeable batteries, smartphone, and TV adapter
- All office visits included
- Hearing technology supplies included (batteries, cleaning accessories, etc.)

The standard cost of the TreatmentFi™ can be customized depending on your hearing and cognitive needs, insurance benefits, and financial situation. Your treatment team will always develop a plan that is right for you!

The medical treatment of hearing loss is associated with a number of physical and cognitive benefits including improvements in quality of life, enhancements in cognitive function, memory recall and attention, and reducing the risk of developing dementia. Additionally, recent reports indicate that the treatment of hearing loss may even slow the *progression* of dementia. Our obligation to our patients is to make treatment accessible, and TreatmentFi™ helps more people make the right decision to treat their hearing loss today.

And don't forget—there are **no hidden costs** in this program. You pay one low monthly fee. Period.

How to Offset the Costs

Use of the TreatmentFi™ program can be customized to meet each patient's needs. Some of the ways that many of my patients cover the low monthly cost is by using their Flexible Spending Account (FSA), using their tax returns, and even writing off the cost of treatment as a medical expense benefit on their tax returns. (Warning: I am not an accountant—and I don't even play one on TV—so always ask your accountant how to best proceed with all tax matters.)

How to use Flexible Spending and eliminate the headache of using it!

Just to make sure we are all on the same page, Flex Spending is accessible through your work benefit package, and it allows you to set aside a certain amount of money per year—TAX-FREE!—to be used towards medical expenses. NeuroTechnology™ and the medical treatment of hearing loss is a medical expense.

Step 1—Sign Up Early!

Perhaps you already follow the "5 P's to Success"—Proper Planning Prevents Poor Performance! But in case you don't, this is one thing you want to plan early for so you can maximize the benefit. Many employees set higher limits than you think on the amount of Flexible Spending dollars you can contribute and access.

I have seen employees with as much as $2,500, and some with even $5,000 in Flex-Spending dollars available to them. Failure to sign up early could cost you more in out-of-pocket medical expenses, especially if your plan is not up and ready before you or a loved one needs to treat his or her hearing loss. If you have a new plan, work with your human resource contact to sign up early for next year in order to maximize your savings.

Step 2—Notify Your Employer of Family Status Changes.

Different employers have different sign-up deadlines for the Flexible Spending plans, but typically at the beginning of the year your employer asks how much money you want to contribute for the year.

The problem with making annual decisions about health care coverage is obvious—life happens and sometimes it's nearly impossible to plan that far ahead! You may apply for a family status change for events such as marriage, birth, divorce, or loss of a spouse's insurance. These are opportunities to add more coverage for hearing loss treatment expenses.

Step 3—Choose Wisely!

Give some thought to calculating how much money to contribute to your flexible plan at work this year—and every year. If you are considering hearing loss treatment for you or a family member, visit your local Excellence In Audiology member-clinic to learn about TreatmentFi™ during initial consultation.

Your patient care coordinator can help you plan exactly how much money you should contribute to help reduce your out-of-pocket costs when it is time to pay for and receive your NeuroTechnology™.

Step 4—Use It or Lose It.

Here's something you may not know—and frankly, it's something which has always puzzled me! If you put more money into your Flex Spending Account than you need or use, by law, you lose the money! Yikes!

You do have three months after the end of the calendar year to submit claims for eligible medical expenses from the previous calendar year. But any money left in your account following this three-month period is forfeited.

QUESTION #19

Does my insurance cover the cost of NeuroTechnology™?

This is a loaded question—and one that I can only answer in general terms because health insurance coverage is a complex ever-changing set of rules, regulations, and specifics that make it impossible to make a blanket statement regarding *your* coverage.

After twenty years of patient care and working with nearly every flavor of insurance coverage, these are my two take-away messages:

1. Nearly every insurance plan, including Medicare, will cover the cost of the comprehensive hearing evaluation.

2. Many patients have some coverage for the cost of treatment (e.g. NeuroTechnology™).

I acknowledge that "nearly every" and "many" are vague terms, but this is the world of insurance we currently live in. I have worked with patients that have $100 of coverage and some with $10,000 in coverage (not that it should ever cost you that much!).

TIP: Do not be afraid to pick up the phone and ask your insurance company point blank: **"Do you cover the cost of treating hearing loss?"** Also, don't be afraid to call back and ask again (you would be shocked how many times our office has called insurance companies seeking this answer only to get a different answer each time we call!). At my office, our Patient Care Coordinators will take the guess work out of the patient's hands and will work directly with the insurance company, and fight with them when needed, to maximize the patient's benefits and coverage.

Bonus Section
Treating Hearing Loss & Your Overall Health

QUESTION #20

What is the research behind the relationship of hearing loss and dementia?

Age-Related Hearing Loss is a progressive and degenerative disorder resulting from the loss of receptor cells (i.e. the hair cells) in the ear. Consequently, there is a significant reduction of the quantity and quality of neural connections from the ear to the brain. This slow-onset disorder can have a significant impact on several key brain areas, including the memory, hearing, speech and language portions of cognitive function. Several key research studies have pointed to the potential links of hearing loss and dementia, including the groundbreaking work from Dr. Lin and his colleagues at Johns Hopkins Medical Center that indicate **hearing loss can increase the risk of Dementia by 200-500%.**

Summary data of relationship of hearing loss and increased risk of developing dementia.

The initial report first published in 2011 by scientists at Johns Hopkins Medical Center and the National Institute on Aging found that individuals with hearing loss (when compared to participants with normal hearing) are at a significantly higher risk of developing dementia as they age. The relationship of hearing loss and increased risk was rather simple: the more hearing loss they had, the higher the likelihood of developing the memory-robbing disease. "A lot of people ignore hearing loss because it's such a slow and insidious process as we age," Dr. Frank Lin (of Johns Hopkins Medical Center) says. "Even if people feel as if they are not affected, we're showing that it may well be a more serious problem."

Three risk factors associated with hearing loss and dementia include Social Isolation, Cerebral Atrophy and Cognitive Overload.

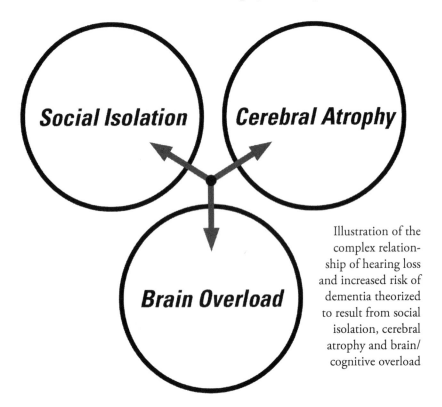

Illustration of the complex relationship of hearing loss and increased risk of dementia theorized to result from social isolation, cerebral atrophy and brain/cognitive overload

1. Social Isolation

The Impact of reduced social and physical activity. Withdrawal from social situations is common in individuals with hearing loss. Many studies cite feelings of embarrassment, fear of making mistakes in conversations, and feeling like you are not part of the conversation as the common rational for individuals with hearing impairment to separate themselves from family, friends and community. This retreat from social activity has even been found in individuals with a mild degree of hearing loss. In addition, individuals with hearing loss are less likely to engage in physical activity. Both increased social isolation and reduced physical activity are strong risk factors for the development of Dementia.

> *Blindness Separates You from Things,*
> *Deafness Separates You from People.*
> — *Helen Keller*

Active Aging: How to Reduce Social Isolation

Active Aging—the process of optimizing opportunities for better health, continuing development of knowledge, and increased security in order to maximize quality of life as you age. The word "active" is used to describe a person's involvement with social, physical, economic, spiritual and civic affairs. We all share the same goal to maintain autonomy and independence as we age, and thus we must rely on preserving the tenants of interdependence (socialization and reliance on family and loved ones) and intergenerational solidarity (maintaining companionship with age-matched peers) to insure active aging.

Both Social Isolation and Depression are risk factors for the development of dementia, and both increase as we age. Being a lifelong learner and staying active is important to maintain a healthy, active brain, and can also reduce your risk of cognitive decline and dementia. Some studies have shown that social activities, larger social networks, and a history of social contact are associated with better cognitive function and reduced risk for cognitive decline.

Tips for Active Aging include:

- Sharing a meal with family and friends 3–5 times per week

- Committing to an aerobics/exercise regiment

- Learning a new hobby each year

- Playing an instrument (or learning a new instrument)

- If you love to read…keep reading (and try to mix up the topics!)

- If you don't read much—try to read a book every other month

- Participating in classes at your local senior center

- Volunteering at a local hospital, shelter, etc.

- Going back to school. Many local state Universities offer free tuition to people over 65!

2. Cerebral Atrophy (AKA Brain Shrinkage)

The association of a shrinking brain, resulting from the loss of neurons, with dementia has been long documented. Even people with MCI (Mild Cognitive Impairment) show signs of cerebral atrophy. In recent years, scientific studies using advanced brain imaging techniques (including fMRI—Functional Magnetic Resonance Imaging) have demonstrated that hearing impairment is associated with accelerated brain atrophy in both the overall brain, as well as even more advanced reductions in volume associated with the memory, hearing, speech and language portions of the brain.

Individuals with hearing loss can experience significant cerebral atrophy. The most significant reduction in cerebral volume occurs in areas involved in memory, hearing, speech and language.

Brain With Hearing Loss   **Brain With Normal Hearing**

Schematic representing the potential cerebral atrophy in an individual with age-related hearing loss.

3. Cognitive Overload (i.e. Working Your Brain Too Hard to Hear)

Hearing loss is not normal, and neither is the excessive strain that it can put on your brain. If you or somebody you love is experiencing hearing loss, you can observe this strain by watching the amount of effort required to follow a conversation. Patients will often joke and say "I need to put my glasses on so I can hear you better." Requiring these extra visual and lip-reading cues may seem a natural way to fill in the missing speech details, but long term these coping mechanisms may have harmful effects on cognitive function.

With hearing loss, the brain is constantly on "overload" trying to fill in the missing pieces, and follow the conversation. I often describe to my patients the taxing effect of hearing loss on brain function by describing the mental effort required to hear "is like driving 60 miles per hour in only second gear."

Increased cognitive load is considered a risk factor for developing dementia. Cognitive load, as measured by pupillometry (i.e. the size of the pupils indicates the amount of mental effort), can quantify how hard your brain is working to follow a conversation. Recent studies have found that individuals who treat their hearing loss do not work as hard to listen (i.e. have a reduced cognitive load) and have as much as a 20% increase in memory recall when following a conversation, even in noisy environments.

QUESTION #21

Can I reduce my increased risk of developing dementia by treating my hearing loss?

As I discuss the relationship of hearing loss and dementia with my patients, each seems to have the same follow up question for me: *"Doc, if I treat my hearing loss, can I prevent or reduce my risk of developing dementia?"*

Thankfully, the data appears to be trending towards a resounding *"**Yes**!"* Recent reports have found a significant positive impact of treating hearing loss on cognitive health.

Treating Hearing Loss and the Impact on Cognitive Function

In a recent study investigating the relationship of treating hearing loss and cognitive function, it was found that current hearing loss treatments can improve brain function in people with hearing loss. It is understood that hearing loss, if left untreated, can lead to emotional and social consequences, reduced job performance, and diminished quality of life. Recently, studies have even shown that untreated hearing loss can interfere with cognitive abilities because so much mental effort is diverted toward understanding speech (i.e. cognitive overload).

The research was aimed at measuring core cognitive functions in subjects in their 50's and 60's beginning hearing loss treatment for the first time. After only two weeks of treatment, cognitive testing began to reveal a significant increase in scores for recalling words in working memory and selective attention tests, and that the processing speed for which participants selected the correct response was significantly faster. In summary: after only a couple of weeks, participants exhibited significant improvement in their cognitive function.

Treating Hearing Loss and the Impact on Risk of Developing Dementia

Since 2011, multiple long-term studies have provided strong evidence that treating hearing loss may eliminate the increased risk of developing dementia. **Dr. Lalwani at Columbia University noted that treating hearing loss...**

> *may offer a simple, yet important, way to prevent or slow the development of dementia by keeping adults with hearing loss engaged in conversation and communication.*

Perhaps the most definitive report comes from the Lancet Commission, which presented a new life-course model documenting potentially modifiable risk factors for dementia. The Commission's report suggests that treating hearing loss is the **single most effective modifiable factor to preventing dementia.** Other modifiable factors include reducing depression, increasing physical activity and reducing social isolation— each of which is positively impacted by treating hearing loss.

QUESTION #22

Can I really expect to be more socially active and engaged once I start treating my hearing loss?

Yes. Throughout this book, I have been providing countless examples of how treating hearing loss can profoundly impact a patient's life and mental health. Frankly, connecting the dots of treating hearing loss to improvements in overall health and personal independence is simple.

If you ask your primary care physician "Doc, what do I need to do to be healthier?", the answer is guaranteed to include reduce stress, increase physical activity, stay socially active and engaged, lose weight, and eat healthy. Treating your hearing loss can help you achieve most of these goals. And achieving these goals is the key to healthy active aging.

There are countless medical studies that find that people who do not treat hearing loss suffer from increased rates of depression, decreased socialization, and decreased physical activity. As an example, the National Council on Aging reported that individuals who do *not* treat hearing loss suffer from depression, anxiety, and decreased social activity. In contrast, individuals who proactively treat their hearing loss find improvements in relationships with family members (spouse, children, grandchildren, etc.), increased self-esteem, and improvements in overall quality of life.

Connecting the Dots of Treating Hearing Loss and Improving Your Life

■ Treating hearing loss can increase physical activity, reduce stress and anxiety, help with losing weight, and ultimately mean living a healthier and more independent lifestyle.

■ Treating hearing loss can increase clarity of speech and the ability to follow conversation in background noise, increase socialization, help reduce the risk of depression, and ultimately mean living a healthier and more independent lifestyle.

■ Treating hearing loss can increase auditory and environmental awareness, decrease the risk of falls, and ultimately mean living a healthier and more independent lifestyle.

■ Treating hearing loss can increase cognitive function, can reduce the increased risk of developing dementia, and ultimately mean living a healthier and more independent lifestyle.

Hearing loss can be isolating for so many people for a multitude of reasons. **But it doesn't have to be.** If you've made it this far through the book, you have come to understand the importance of treating hearing loss and taking care of your brain—and how these two are connected.

I wish you luck and happiness as you embark on the journey of treating hearing loss, restoring clarity, increasing independence, and keeping a healthy and fit brain!

HEARING TREATMENT

IMPROVED OVERALL HEALTH

Epilogue

You Had Questions and I Hope I've Provided Answers

So, there you have it! Twenty-two of my patients' most popular questions answered (for your convenience I've included a handy FAQ directly after this epilogue that summarizes most, if not all, of the questions we've just covered. Consider it a handy "quick reference" of sorts).

The fact is no book can ever answer EVERY question for every patient. Every case is unique, just as every patient with hearing loss that I treat is different. What I've tried to do is provide you with the basics and, hopefully, the confidence you'll need to ask further questions of your own hearing care specialist when the time comes.

This is your hearing, your brain, and your overall health we are talking about here; never be afraid to insist on being heard and having your questions answered by your clinician. Now that you're armed with the answers for today's most frequently asked audiology questions, you can finally make the right decision for you or a loved one when embarking on the journey of medical treatment for hearing loss.

When you are ready to take the next step to improve your life, your cognitive function, and your hearing health, please visit:

ExcellenceInAudiology.com
or call **(352) 269-4818**
to Schedule a Consultation

faqs

A Resource Guide
of Frequently
Asked Questions
& Terminology

What might happen if I wait to treat my hearing loss?

Even mild hearing loss can be a major problem for a number of reasons. Hearing loss can increase the risk of developing dementia and is correlated with several other major diseases including diabetes, coronary disease, and kidney disease. Early treatment also improves the treatment prognosis and expected outcomes.

Who are some famous people who've invested in treating their hearing loss with technology?

The list is quite long! A (much) abbreviated list includes presidents Reagan, Clinton, and George H.W. Bush, and other celebrities and famous athletes including Huey Lewis, Lou Ferrigno, William Shatner, Pete Townshend, Whoopi Goldberg, Derrick Coleman, Congressman Jim Ryun, Phil Collins, and Brian Kerwin.

Will I be able to afford NeuroTechnology™?

Yes. TreatmentFi™ provides the highest level of hearing health care to meet your hearing loss and cognitive needs, all at an affordable, set, low, monthly price!

Will being fit with NeuroTechnology™ be painful or obvious to others?

No and no. Advances in miniaturization of technology have helped develop the most light-weight, discrete, and sometimes completely invisible technology ever used to treat hearing loss.

Will I have to miss work or other social activities once fit with NeuroTechnology™?

The initial comprehensive evaluation and treatment procedures will take between one to one and a half hours. Follow-up visits after that will only take between fifteen to thirty minutes. Patients walk out of the office after the first appointment and go about their lives…only now they can hear *MUCH* better!

Is it really such a big deal if I don't treat my hearing loss?

Yes. Too many people believe that their hearing loss is "normal for their age." There is no such thing as "normal" or "age-corrected" hearing loss. Hearing loss is a progressive degenerative disorder that will continue to negatively impact your life and cognition the longer it goes untreated.

What are some of the warning signs that I may have hearing loss?

Early symptoms of hearing loss include difficulty following conversation in background noise, experiencing tinnitus (ringing in the ears), having to turn up the TV louder than others need it, asking people to repeat often, finding yourself needing to read lips to hear better, difficulty understanding on the phone, and your family bugging you about getting help.

What kind of side-effects can result from NOT treating my hearing loss?

Untreated hearing loss is implicated in increased risk of falls, development of dementia, diabetes, coronary disease, depression, as well as increased stress and reduced physical activity.

Why should I choose a specialist to treat my hearing loss?

Hearing loss is a major medical condition and has been listed as the **third most common** medical disorder impacting seniors. Unfortunately, loopholes in many state and federal laws allow for traditional hearing aids to be sold in retail establishments, including some of the big-box discount stores. These traditional hearing aids are most often older models and are only designed to amplify sound.

NeuroTechnology™, designed to treat the cognitive aspects of hearing loss, is the "gold-standard" and considered "best practices" by audiologists and board-certified specialists in private practice audiology clinics.

How do I know if my hearing care provider is a Doctor of Audiology?

This is typically pretty easy to figure out by searching the internet or even calling the office. I've never been bothered by a patient calling to confirm my credentials prior to his or her arrival—in fact, I believe this shows a proper amount of due diligence on the part of the patient and a true investment in his or her hearing health care. Most states will also provide a list or search tool online to find licensed and certified providers.

What is a Patient Care Coordinator?

During your initial consultation(s), you will usually be assigned a patient contact person—we call this person a Patient Care Coordinator in our office—with whom to schedule appointments, confer with for rescheduling, and, of course, help you get answers to any and all questions you may have at any point in the process.

Why are follow-up visits important?

These are wonderful opportunities to ask questions you may have missed the first time, get further details from your specialist, and bring a family member to learn about your diagnosis and treatment plan.

Why is early treatment so important?

Since we recommend adults fifty and older to have a comprehensive hearing evaluation, we have coined the term "Ears and Rears"! This is meant to remind people to add hearing to their list of medical appointments once they turn fifty. At fifty, if the patient is found to have hearing loss, it is critical to start treatment early to avoid some of the devastating consequences of untreated hearing loss. Alternatively, if the patient has normal hearing, a baseline will be established and used for comparison at follow-up appointments.

What if I don't believe in early treatment of age-related hearing loss?

Unfortunately, for many patients it takes nearly seven years for them to admit they have hearing loss (or to succumb to pressure from family members) and start treatment. By this time, the hearing loss will typically be at a moderate degree or beyond and, in some cases, treatment outcomes can be negatively impacted. To assure a positive prognosis and improved treatment outcomes, hearing loss must be caught early and treated early to maintain positive connections to the brain. *"Catch it early and treat it early!"*

What is sensorineural hearing loss?

Sensorineural hearing loss (SNHL) is a hearing impairment that results from damage to, or dysfunction of, the inner ear (cochlear) and/or the auditory nervous system. Age-related hearing loss is a form of sensorineural hearing loss.

What is a conductive hearing loss?

Conductive hearing loss (CHL) is a hearing impairment that results from damage to, or dysfunction of, the outer ear (pinna and ear canal) and/or the middle ear (the eardrum or ossicles—hammer, anvil and stirrup). In some cases of CHL, surgical intervention can help restore hearing function.

What is a processing disorder?

Hearing loss is often defined in terms of the amount of lost volume that results from either a SNHL or a CHL. However, many patients, even those with normal hearing levels, can have a processing disorder that will limit their ability to understand and follow speech in background noise. The noise cancellation feature in NeuroTechnology™ provides significant benefit by reducing background noise and enhancing speech—even for those with normal hearing.

Should I bring a family member with me to my appointment(s)?

I answer this with a decisive **YES**. Your hearing loss not only impacts you but also everybody around you. I have always encouraged every patient to bring a spouse or a loved one to every appointment so he or she can help me, and the patient, better understand the daily impact of hearing loss on everybody's life.

What is NeuroTechnology™?

In recent years, traditional hearing aids, which simply make sounds louder, have been phased out and replaced with NeuroTechnology™. The significant cognitive benefits to NeuroTechnology™ include: *binaural processing* (two ears working together), *sound orientation* (ability to detect the source of incoming sounds with increased accuracy), *enhanced clarity of voices* (even soft speakers), automatic *adaptation to environment* (no more pushing buttons and adjusting volume), and *noise-cancellation* filtering of background noise to enhance hearing conversation in noisy environments (hearing better in crowded rooms, restaurants, etc.).

What is the primary benefit of NeuroTechnology™?

This answer is outlined in greater detail throughout the book. In summary, recent reports find that NeuroTechnology™ and the treatment of hearing loss can significantly improve quality of life, reduce the risk of developing dementia, and offer an increase in cognitive function. Yes, all of this can be achieved by treating your hearing loss.

How do I get started with NeuroTechnology™?

It's simple: Request an appointment with the local audiology clinic that sent you this book, or visit *www.ExcellenceinAudiology.org* to find a member-clinic in your area. Most clinics will offer a free initial consultation to see if you are a good candidate for hearing loss treatment.

Is getting traditional hearing aids still effective treatment for hearing loss?

For the majority of patients, traditional hearing aids will not effectively treat hearing loss or the symptoms of hearing loss, including tinnitus. Traditional hearing aids are volume-enhancing devices that may help certain people in very limited environments (e.g. conversing one-on-one in a room with *no* background noise). For patients needing to follow conversation in dynamic environments (e.g. sitting at a dinner table with family and friends, going out to a restaurant, sitting in a lecture hall or a place of worship, playing cards with others, etc.), NeuroTechnology™ will restore clarity and enhance speech even in background noise.

Can I use my insurance benefit and Flex-Spending with TreatmentFi™?

Yes. TreatmentFi™ is customized to meet your hearing, cognitive, and financial needs. With this program, any insurance benefit you may have can be deducted from your monthly payment. In addition, payment for the treatment of hearing loss can be paid for through the use of a Flexible Spending Account set up at your employer.

What if I need an emergency appointment before or after office hours?

(This answer is a bit longer than most because of the seriousness of some audiology emergencies)

Audiology emergencies most often fall in to one of two categories:

Sudden change in hearing

While rare, a sudden change in hearing can occur. This medical condition, known as *sudden-onset sensorineural hearing loss*, may occur in one, or both (even more rare), ears and is often associated with a virus (and sometimes occurs in tandem with an upper respiratory infection).

There is varying data on successful treatment protocols for this disorder; regardless, the key to potentially recovering hearing function requires seeking medical attention within 24–48 hours of initial symptoms.

Emergency related to the NeuroTechnology™

Broken or "non-functioning devices" may occur from time to time during your treatment. If there is any disturbance, such as lost domes, tight speaker wires, or irritation, call your hearing care provider's office as soon as possible to have them evaluate the urgency of the problem and schedule you to be seen accordingly. In the interim, here are helpful hints to remedy some of the problems that you may encounter until you can be seen in the office:

- If a device is itching your ear, use some ear lotion included in your treatment package.
- A device causing feedback or "squealing" can generally be worn until you are seen by our team. Call the office as soon as you notice this feedback or squealing so that we can schedule you to make a prescription change.

■ A dome, earmold, or removable device that is not fitting well, is not to be worn until it can be properly adjusted at the office. Call the office as soon as possible to have your specialists make the adjustment for comfort and fit.

If you are experiencing an audiology emergency that can't wait for regular office hours, most audiology offices have a special number to call either before or after business hours. If you can wait until the office is open, most offices will have special emergency appointments set aside each day to help in these situations.

Can NeuroTechnology™ get wet?

Unlike traditional hearing aids that had no moisture resistance, most of today's NeuroTechnology™ comes with an IP57 rating for dust and moisture resistance. In lay terms, the "IP" stands for International Protection Rating and the "5" indicates the unit is Dust Protected (highest score is a 6 on this scale) and the "7" indicates the unit can be immersed in up to one meter of water (that is over three feet!). With that said—we continue to direct patients to not swim or bathe with their NeuroTechnology™.

Should I sleep with my NeuroTechnology™?

It is recommended to *not* sleep with your NeuroTechnology™ for three reasons:

1. Give your ear a rest—sleeping with the unit can cause discomfort to the pinna and side of the head.

2. It is easier for the unit to fall out when tossing and turning in bed and may get lost.

3. It will wear out the batteries in half the time of their intended lifespan if used 24 hours per day.

However, I do have patients that sleep with their NeuroTechnology™ for safety and personal reasons.

How do I regularly clean my NeuroTechnology™?

Like with cleaning your home…clean it a little each day and it won't become such a mess! Your specialist will help you understand daily and monthly routines for maintaining your NeuroTechnology™ at home. Use a lint free cloth and brush (typically provided at your first treatment appointment) to wipe down the unit every day. This will help prevent oils from the skin, dandruff, earwax, and other environmental dust from clogging the microphones and speaker over time. I also encourage my patients to change the "parts" once a month. This includes wax filters (designed to prevent earwax from entering the unit), domes (designed to securely hold the unit in the ear) and microphone filters (included on some NeuroTechnology™ options).

Bibliography
The Science Behind Everything You Read In This Book

This book is the result of my 20+ years in hearing health care. In this time, I have amassed information from my research, reading of scientific publications, in the classroom (as student and teacher), and from directly interacting with patients' and their loved ones. Below is a list of references that helped me put together this book and present the information to you in a succinct manner. You can access these manuscripts on Google Scholar and/or Pubmed.

"Active Ageing: A Policy Framework." *The Aging Male* 5, no. 1 (2002), 1-37.

Adult Cognition and Hearing Aids. U of Canterbury. Communication Disorders, 2015.

Agmon, Maayan, Limor Lavie, and Michail Doumas. "The Association between Hearing Loss, Postural Control, and Mobility in Older Adults: A Systematic Review." *Journal of the American Academy of Audiology* 28, no. 6 (2017), 575-588.

"Association of Hearing Impairment and Subsequent Driving Mobility in Older Adults." *The Gerontologist* 55, no. Suppl_2 (2015), 137-138.

Bainbridge, Kathleen E., Howard J. Hoffman, and Catherine C. Cowie. "Diabetes and Hearing Impairment in the United States: Audiometric Evidence from the National Health and Nutrition Examination Survey, 1999 to 2004." *Annals of Internal Medicine* 149, no. 1 (2008), 1.

Bassuk, Shari S., Thomas A. Glass, and Lisa F. Berkman. "Social Disengagement and Incident Cognitive Decline in Community-Dwelling Elderly Persons." *Annals of Internal Medicine* 131, no. 3 (1999), 165.

Bernabei, Roberto, Ubaldo Bonuccelli, Stefania Maggi, Alessandra Marengoni, Alessandro Martini, Maurizio Memo, Sergio Pecorelli, Andrea P. Peracino, Nicola Quaranta, and Roberto Stella. "Hearing loss and cognitive decline in older adults: questions and answers." *Aging Clinical and Experimental Research* 26, no. 6 (2014), 567-573.

Burns, Elizabeth R., Judy A. Stevens, and Robin Lee. "The direct costs of fatal and non-fatal falls among older adults — United States." *Journal of Safety Research* 58 (2016), 99-103.

Cardin, Velia. "Effects of Aging and Adult-Onset Hearing Loss on Cortical Auditory Regions." *Frontiers in Neuroscience* 10 (2016).

Cass, SP. "Alzheimer's Disease and Exercise: A Literature Review." *Curr. Sports Med. Rep*, February 16, 2017.

Chen, David S., Dane J. Genther, Joshua Betz, and Frank R. Lin. "Association Between Hearing Impairment and Self-Reported Difficulty in Physical Functioning." *Journal of the American Geriatrics Society* 62, no. 5 (2014), 850-856.

Chia, Ee-Munn, Jie J. Wang, Elena Rochtchina, Robert R. Cumming, Philip Newall, and Paul Mitchell. "Hearing Impairment and Health-Related Quality of Life: The Blue Mountains Hearing Study." *Ear and Hearing* 28, no. 2 (2007), 187-195.

Collins, John G. "Prevalence of Selected Chronic Conditions: United States, 1983-85." *PsycEXTRA Dataset* (n.d.).

Davidson, JGS. "Older Adults With a Combination of Vision and Hearing Impairment Experience Higher Rates of Cognitive Impairment, Functional Dependence, and Worse Outcomes Across a Set of Quality Indicators." Last modified August 1, 2017.

De Leon, M. J., S. DeSanti, R. Zinkowski, P. D. Mehta, D. Pratico, S. Segal, C. Clark, D. Kerkman, J. DeBernardis, and J. Li. "MRI and CSF studies in the early diagnosis of Alzheimer's disease." *Journal of Internal Medicine* 256, no. 3 (2004), 205-223.

Deal, Jennifer A., Josh Betz, Kristine Yaffe, Tamara Harris, Elizabeth Purchase-Helzner, Suzanne Satterfield, Sheila Pratt, Nandini Govil, Eleanor M. Simonsick, and Frank R. Lin. "Hearing Impairment and Incident Dementia and Cognitive Decline in Older Adults: The Health ABC Study." *The Journals of Gerontology Series A: Biological Sciences and Medical Sciences*, 2016, glw069.

"Dementia Prevention, Intervention, and Care." *Lancet*, July 19, 2017.

Desjardins, Jamie L. "Analysis of Performance on Cognitive Test Measures Before, During, and After 6 Months of Hearing Aid Use: A Single-Subject Experimental Design." *American Journal of Audiology* 25, no. 2 (2016), 127.

Ferreira, Lidiane M., Alberto N. Ramos, and Eveline P. Mendes. "Characterization of tinnitus in the elderly and its possible related disorders." *Brazilian Journal of Otorhinolaryngology* 75, no. 2 (2009), 249-255.

Genther, Dane J., Joshua Betz, Sheila Pratt, Kathryn R. Martin, Tamara B. Harris, Suzanne Satterfield, Douglas C. Bauer, Anne B. Newman, Eleanor M. Simonsick, and Frank R. Lin. "Association Between Hearing Impairment and Risk of Hospitalization in Older Adults." *Journal of the American Geriatrics Society* 63, no. 6 (2015), 1146-1152.

Gibrin, PC, AN Ramos Junior, and EP Mendes. "Prevalence of Tinnitus Complaints and Probable Association with Hearing Loss, Diabetes Mellitus and Hypertension in Elderly." *Codas*, 2013.

Gispen, Fiona E., David S. Chen, Dane J. Genther, and Frank R. Lin. "Association Between Hearing Impairment and Lower Levels of Physical Activity in Older Adults." *Journal of the American Geriatrics Society* 62, no. 8 (2014), 1427-1433.

Govender, SM, CD Govender, and G. Matthews. "Cochlear Function in Patients with Chronic Kidney Disease." *South African/Commun Diord*, December 2013.

Haan, Mary N. "Can Social Engagement Prevent Cognitive Decline in Old Age?" *Annals of Internal Medicine* 131, no. 3 (1999), 220.

"Hearing Impairment and Frailty in English Community-Dwelling Older Adults: A 4-Year Follow-Up Study." *The Gerontologist* 56, no. Suppl_3 (2016), 319-319.

"Hearing Loss and Cognitive Decline in Older Adults." *JAMA Internal Medicine*, February 25, 2013.

"The Impact of Hearing Loss on Quality of Life in Older Adults." *Gerontologist*, October 2003.

"The Impact of Hearing Loss on quality of Life in Older Adults." *Gerontologist*, October 2003.

"An Introduction to MarkeTrak IX: A New Baseline for the Hearing Aid Market." *Hearing Review*, May 15, 2015.

Jacoby, R., and R. Levy. "CT Scanning and the Investigation of Dementia: A Review." *J.R. Soc. Med*, May 1980.

Jamaldeen, Jishana, Aneesh Basheer, Akhil Sarma, and Ravichandran Kandasamy. "Prevalence and patterns of hearing loss among chronic kidney disease patients undergoing haemodialysis." *australasian medical journal*, 2015, 41-46.

Kamil, Rebecca J., Lingsheng Li, and Frank R. Lin. "Association between Hearing Impairment and Frailty in Older Adults." *Journal of the American Geriatrics Society* 62, no. 6 (2014), 1186-1188.

Kelley, Amy S., Kathleen McGarry, Rebecca Gorges, and Jonathan S. Skinner. "The Burden of Health Care Costs for Patients With Dementia in the Last 5 Years of Life." *Annals of Internal Medicine* 163, no. 10 (2015), 729.

Kochkin, Sergei. "MarkeTrak VII." *The Hearing Journal* 60, no. 4 (2007), 24-51.

Lambert, Justin, Rouzbeh Ghadry-Tavi, Kate Knuff, Marc Jutras, Jodi Siever, Paul Mick, Carolyn Roque, Gareth Jones, Jonathan Little, and Harry Miller. "Targeting functional fitness, hearing and health-related quality of life in older adults with hearing loss: Walk, Talk 'n' Listen, study protocol for a pilot randomized controlled trial." *Trials* 18, no. 1 (2017).

Le Goff, Nicolas, Dorothea Wendt, Thomas Lunner, and Elaine Ng. "Opn Clinical Evidence. Oticon White Paper." 2016.

Lin, F.R., L. Ferrucci, Y. An, J.O. Goh, Jimit Doshi, E.J. Metter, C. Davatzikos, M.A. Kraut, and S.M. Resnick. "Association of hearing impairment with brain volume changes in older adults." *NeuroImage* 90 (2014), 84-92.

Lin, Frank R. "Hearing Loss Prevalence in the United States." *Archives of Internal Medicine*171, no. 20 (2011), 1851.

Lin, Frank R. "Hearing Loss and Falls Among Older Adults in the United States." *Archives of Internal Medicine* 172, no. 4 (2012), 369.

Lin, Frank R., E. J. Metter, Richard J. O'Brien, Susan M. Resnick, Alan B. Zonderman, and Luigi Ferrucci. "Hearing Loss and Incident Dementia." *Archives of Neurology* 68, no. 2 (2011).

Martini, Alessandro, Alessandro Castiglione, Roberto Bovo, Antonino Vallesi, and Carlo Gabelli. "Aging, Cognitive Load, Dementia and Hearing Loss." *Audiology and Neurotology* 19, no. 1 (2014), 2-5.

Meister, Hartmut, Stefan Schreitmüller, Magdalene Ortmann, Sebastian Rählmann, and Martin Walger. "Effects of Hearing Loss and Cognitive Load on Speech Recognition with Competing Talkers." *Frontiers in Psychology* 7 (2016).

Melse-Boonstra, Alida, and Ian Mackenzie. "Iodine deficiency, thyroid function and hearing deficit: a review." *Nutrition Research Reviews* 26, no. 02 (2013), 110-117.

Meyerhoff, William L. "The Thyroid and Audition." *The Laryngoscope* 86, no. 4 (1976), 483-489.

Miyawaki, Christina E., E. D. Bouldin, G. S. Kumar, and L. C. McGuire. "Associations between physical activity and cognitive functioning among middle-aged and older adults." *The journal of nutrition, health & aging* 21, no. 6 (2016), 637-647.

Mulrow, Cynthia D., Christine Aguilar, James E. Endicott, Ramon Velez, Michael R. Tuley, Walter S. Charlip, and Judith A. Hill. "Association Between Hearing Impairment and the Quality of Life of Elderly Individuals." *Journal of the American Geriatrics Society* 38, no. 1 (1990), 45-50.

Oh, Esther, Frank Lin, and Sara Mamo. "Enhancing Communication in Adults with Dementia and Age-Related Hearing Loss." *Seminars in Hearing* 38, no. 02 (2017), 177-183.

Palmer, Andrew D., Jason T. Newsom, and Karen S. Rook. "How does difficulty communicating affect the social relationships of older adults? An exploration using data from a national survey." *Journal of Communication Disorders* 62 (2016), 131-146.

Popelka, Michael M., Karen J. Cruickshanks, Terry L. Wiley, Theodore S. Tweed, Barbara E. Klein, and Ronald Klein. "Low Prevalence of Hearing Aid Use Among Older Adults with Hearing Loss: The Epidemiology of Hearing Loss Study." *Journal of the American Geriatrics Society* 46, no. 9 (1998), 1075-1078.

Qian, Z. J., Peter D. Chang, Gul Moonis, and Anil K. Lalwani. "A novel method of quantifying brain atrophy associated with age-related hearing loss." *NeuroImage: Clinical* 16 (2017), 205-209.

Qian, Zhen J., Kapil Wattamwar, Francesco F. Caruana, Jenna Otter, Matthew J. Leskowitz, Barbara Siedlecki, Jaclyn B. Spitzer, and Anil K. Lalwani. "Hearing Aid Use is Associated with Better Mini-Mental State Exam Performance." *The American Journal of Geriatric Psychiatry* 24, no. 9 (2016), 694-702.

Ryu, Nam-Gyu, Il J. Moon, Hayoung Byun, Sun H. Jin, Heesung Park, Kyu-Sun Jang, and Yang-Sun Cho. "Clinical effectiveness of wireless CROS (contralateral routing of offside signals) hearing aids." *European Archives of Oto-Rhino-Laryngology* 272, no. 9 (2014), 2213-2219.

Seimetz, Bruna, Adriane Teixeira, Leticia Rosito, Leticia Flores, Carlos Pappen, and Celso Dall'igna. "Pitch and Loudness Tinnitus in Individuals with Presbycusis." *International Archives of Otorhinolaryngology* 20, no. 04 (2016), 321-326.

Sindhusake, Doungkamol, Paul Mitchell, Philip Newall, Maryanne Golding, Elena Rochtchina, and George Rubin. "Prevalence and characteristics of tinnitus in older adults: the Blue Mountains Hearing Study: Prevalencia y características del acúfeno en adultos mayores: el Estudio de Audición Blue Mountains." *International Journal of Audiology* 42, no. 5 (2003), 289-294.

Snapp, Hillary A., Fred D. Holt, Xuezhong Liu, and Suhrud M. Rajguru. "Comparison of Speech-in-Noise and Localization Benefits in Unilateral Hearing Loss Subjects Using Contralateral Routing of Signal Hearing Aids or Bone-Anchored Implants." *Otology & Neurotology* 38, no. 1 (2017), 11-18.

"Social Isolation in Community-Dwelling Seniors: An Evidence-Based Analysis." *Health Quality Ontario*, August 2008.

Spulber, Gabriela, Eini Niskanen, Stuart MacDonald, Oded Smilovici, Kewei Chen, Eric M. Reiman, Anne M. Jauhiainen, Merja Hallikainen, Susanna Tervo, and Lars-Olof Wahlund. "Whole brain atrophy rate predicts progression from MCI to Alzheimer's disease." *Neurobiology of Aging* 31, no. 9 (2010), 1601-1605.

Su, Peijen, Chih-Chao Hsu, Hung-Ching Lin, Wei-Shin Huang, Tsung-Lin Yang, Wei-Ting Hsu, Cheng-Li Lin, Chung-Yi Hsu, Kuang-Hsi Chang, and Yi-Chao Hsu. "Age-related hearing loss and dementia: a 10-year national population-based study." *European Archives of Oto-Rhino-Laryngology* 274, no. 5 (2017), 2327-2334.

Vignesh, S. S., V. Jaya, Anand Moses, and A. Muraleedharan. "Identifying Early Onset of Hearing Loss in Young Adults With Diabetes Mellitus Type 2 Using High Frequency Audiometry." *Indian Journal of Otolaryngology and Head & Neck Surgery* 67, no. 3 (2014), 234-237.

Weinstein, Barbara E. *Hearing Impairment and Social Isolation in the Elderly*. publisher not identified, 1980.

Yates, J.A., L. Clare, and B. Woods. "You've Got a Friend in Me: Can Social Engagement Mediate the Relationship Between Mood and MCI?" *Innovation in Aging* 1, no. suppl_1 (2017), 1179-1179.

Yates, Jennifer A., Linda Clare, and Robert T. Woods. "What is the Relationship between Health, Mood, and Mild Cognitive Impairment?" *Journal of Alzheimer's Disease* 55, no. 3 (2016), 1183-1193.

Zheng, Yuqiu, Shengnuo Fan, Wang Liao, Wenli Fang, Songhua Xiao, and Jun Liu. "Hearing impairment and risk of Alzheimer's disease: a meta-analysis of prospective cohort studies." *Neurological Sciences* 38, no. 2 (2016), 233-239.

If you read this book, chances are that you or a family member are struggling to deal with impact of hearing loss on your social, physical, and mental well-being. By now I hope you have come to understand the negative impact of untreated hearing loss on overall quality of life and cognitive function.

We thank you for taking your hearing healthcare seriously and for allowing us to provide the education necessary for you to make an informed decision about medically treating your hearing loss.

When you are ready to take the next step to improve your life, your cognitive function, and your hearing health, please visit:

ExcellenceInAudiology.com
or call **(352) 269-4818**
to Schedule a Consultation

EXCELLENCE™
IN AUDIOLOGY

Made in the USA
Columbia, SC
23 January 2020

87031994R00074